Thanks for choosing this book. I wish you a good read and, if you like, leave a short review on Amazon.

Amy

SIRTFOOD DIET:

a Complete Beginner's Guide to Lose Weight,

Boost Metabolism,

Gain Energy, and Feel Great

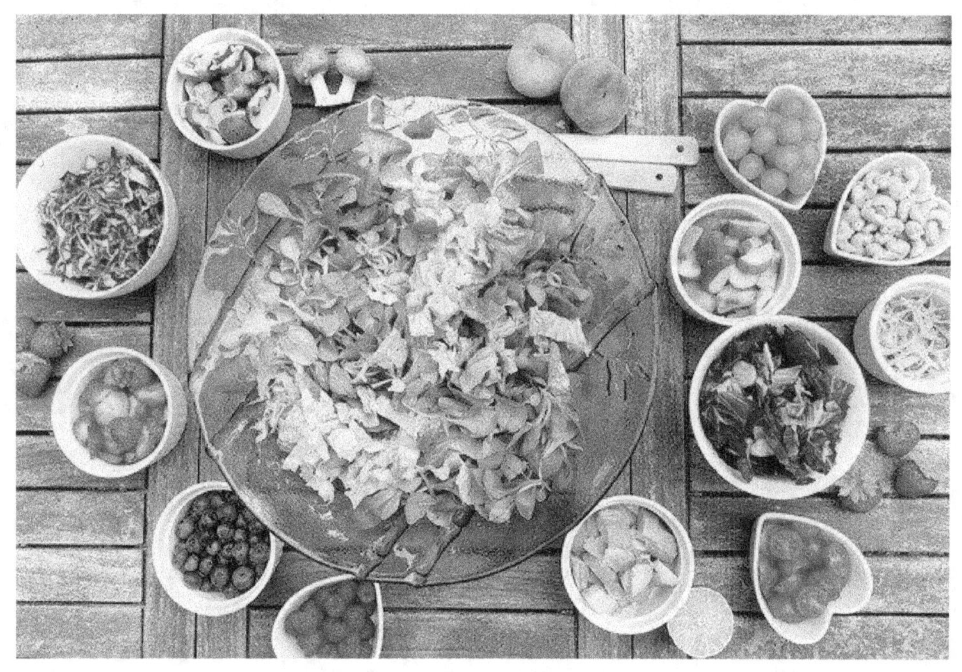

By Amy Cook

Table of Contents

Introduction

For so many years, a ton of several diets has been studied and practiced by many people to achieve weight loss, better health, and to set restrictions according to one's dietary needs. Some diets may work, and some may not, and it's very challenging for a person to abide and make changes every now then just looking for a diet that will be effective for them. You'll discover the new diet sensation recognized internationally that will aid a person to shed 7 pounds in 7 days while still having lasting energy and consuming foods they love.

The sirtfood diet is developed based on the fact that some foods are capable of activating *sirtuins* in your body. The Sirtfood Diet was formed by nutrition experts Aiden Goggins and Glen Matten. They were so interested in the possibilities of Sirtfoods, and they created a diet based around maximizing Sirtfood intake and mild calorie restriction.

Sirtuins are also fondly called skinny genes, which are particular proteins to obtain a variety of benefits, which range from shielding cells in your body from inflammation to reversing aging. Through the activation of sirtuins, the storage of fat will be shut off, and the body will enter its survival mode. In this survival mode, fat burning is stimulated, and the genes drawn in the rejuvenation and repair of the cells are activated, as mentioned a while ago, which will then result in loss of weight and improved resistance to sickness. Like any other diet, the improper practice of diet will lead to irritability, hunger, loss of muscle, and fatigue. That is why having the proper knowledge in all aspects of the diet is needed to prevent such adverse effects.

There's no denying that sirtfoods benefit you. They are frequently high in nutrients and complete healthy plant compounds. It is made to be useful for the long term and makes you healthy for life. Moreover, research studies have associated many of the foods recommended on the Sirtfood Diet with health advantages. Apart from that, one can't deny that sirtfood ingredients are, in fact, delicious, which will make one satisfied. This makes it very beneficial for the one doing the diet, as they get the benefits and at the same time have the satisfaction of eating tasty foods.

For example, consuming moderate amounts of dark chocolate with high cocoa content might decrease the danger of cardiovascular disease and assistance fight inflammation. Drinking green tea might reduce the risk of stroke and diabetes and help lower high blood pressure. And turmeric has anti-inflammatory properties that have beneficial impacts on the body in general and may even secure against chronic, inflammation-related illness).

The bulk of sirtfoods have demonstrated health benefits in people. And throughout fasting or calorie limitation, sirtuin proteins inform the body to burn more fat for energy and improve insulin level of sensitivity. Without further ado, let's learn how we can apply this diet!

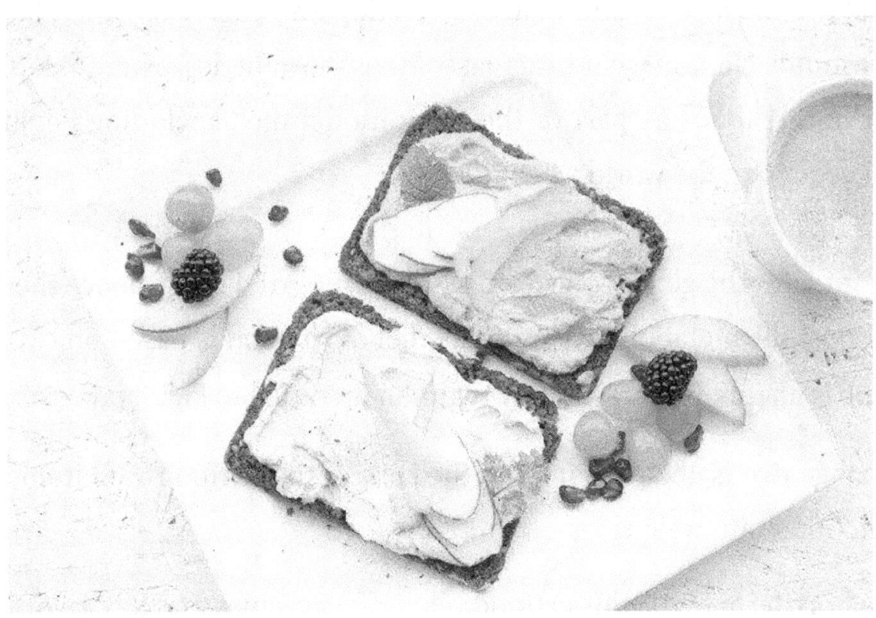

Chapter 1

What is The Sirt Food Diet/ VIP Diet?

Any diet that professes to turn on your "thin qualities" makes sure to knock some people's socks off—and undoubtedly set off your B.S. locator. However, that is actually what the Sirtfood Diet professes to do.

The founders of the sirtfood diet are Aidan Goggin's and glen matte, both professional nutritionists who have succeeded in harnessing the influence of 'sirtfood' research to build a groundbreaking diet.

Diet research is all about these sirtfoods, a collection of recently identified daily plant foods rich in a chemical compound known as 'sirtuin' activators. These sirtuin activators are a kind of protein that turns into the body's 'skinny gene' pathway. These slender pathways are the same ones that are most often stimulated by fasting and exercise, which help the body lose weight, increase muscle mass, and increase fitness. Countries where people already eat a large number of Sirt foods as part of their traditional diet, including Japan and Italy, are regularly ranked among the world's healthiest.

Sirtfood stimulates the genes of sirtuin, which is reported to influence the body's ability to burn fat and boost the metabolic system. The diet of sirtfood is based on two stages;

- Step one is an intensive seven-day regimen intended to kick-start extreme weight loss.

- Then, stage two is about adding up the sum of the sirtfood-rich items in your regular meals to maintain weight loss.

Like other short-term diets, the sirtfood plan offers recipes and advice on how to keep the weight you lose within the first week while attempting to adopt sirtfood as part of a healthy and balanced lifestyle.

Dieters consume two natural drinks a day for the first three days, including spinach, celery, rocket, parsley, lemon, and green tea, and eat one meal.

For example, with garlic, rice, kale curry, pomegranate, or sesame-glazed tofu, it may be something like turkey escalope if you're vegetarian. Both of them made up of ingredients rich in sirtfood. You can also get 15-20 g of dark chocolate after dinner if you have a sweet tooth. You'll have two drinks and two dinners a day for the second half of the first week, with the same recipes as the early three days.

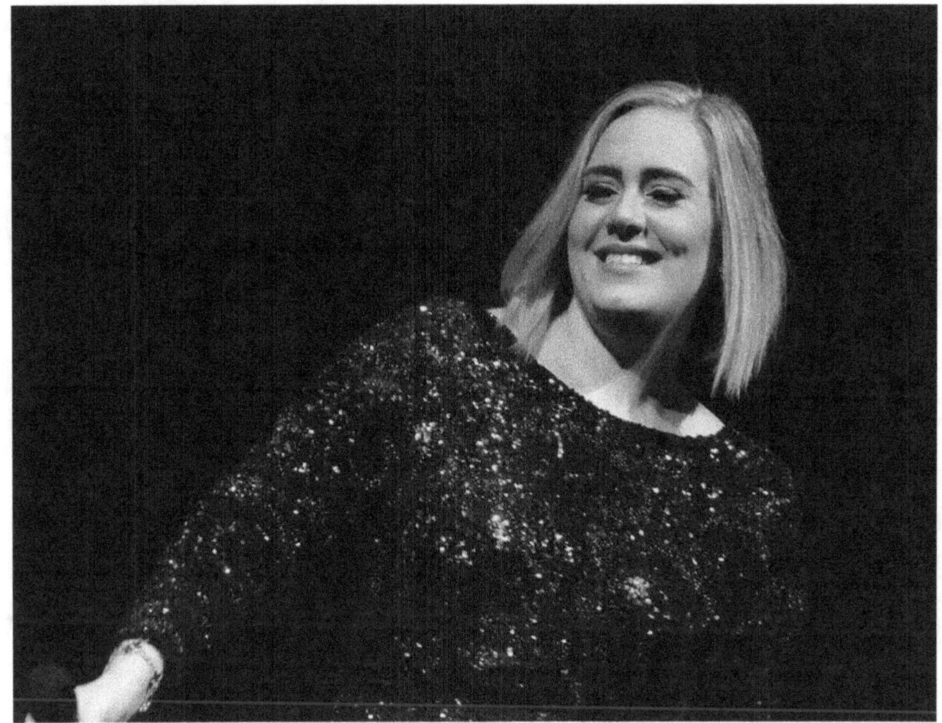

Photo by Kristopher Harris (CC BY 2.0)

The emphasis shifts to eating 'normally' again after the initial fasting stage; however, high the consumption of balanced sirt foods may be. While the initial step of juicing and fasting is just unusual for someone who might want to turn a few pounds immediately, the general approach of sirtfood's diet is to incorporate healthy foods into your diet to improve your well-being and strengthen your immune system over time. So, while the first seven days seem to be hardcore, the longer-term plan works for everyone. You will start burning fat when you enjoy your daily treats by focusing on adding rich sirtfood ingredients to your daily meals.

The biggest plus is that this lifestyle actively promotes red wine, dark chocolate, and coffee, and you don't always say that! The compounds that make up our favorite treats are abundant in sirtuin actuators. Although, of course, eating a kale smoothie, accompanied by a whole bar of greens and blacks, doesn't mean losing your pounds. It's all in balance. Participants never get hungry – which suggests that it's perfect for someone who can't get through a regular cleaning day without feeling like they're going to die because they don't have a vast mac right away.

The first week of the plan is very intense. Days one to three are the most concentrated with a maximum calorie intake of 1000 – a mixture of three drinks and one dinner. Day four to seven is marginally leniency, with an average calorie of 1,500 calories per day.
Sirtfood is almost all healthy choices, and due to its anti-inflammatory and antioxidant properties, it can even produce some health benefits. Yet eating only a chosen list of healthy foods cannot satisfy all of one's body's needed nutrients. Sirtfood diet is not necessarily restrictive and does not offer any definite health benefits over any other food. Also, it is not usually recommended to consume just 1,000 calories without the guidance of a specialist.

For many people, even eating 1500 calories a day is overly restrictive. Consuming up to three green juices daily is also required in the diet. While liquids can be a good source of minerals and vitamins, they are likewise a source of sugar and has hardly any of the nutritious fibers made by whole vegetables and fruits.

What's more, all-day juice sipping is not a good thing for both your teeth and sugar levels of blood. Also, due to the reason that the diet has limitations in calories and food choices, nutrients, minerals, and vitamins are more than necessary, especially during the primary stage.

This diet may be challenging to maintain for three weeks due to low-calorie levels and restrictive food choices. Connect this to the expensive cost of purchasing a juicer, a book, and other odd and expensive items, as well as the time cost of cooking various foods and juices. This lifestyle is unfeasible and impractical for a few.

Although the first step of the sirtfood diet is tiny in calories and incomplete, nutrition-wise, due to the limited duration of the menu, there are no particular safety issues for a healthy, stable person. However, reducing calories and only drinking juice during the initial stages of the diet can cause adverse levels of blood sugar for those with diabetes.

However, also a healthy person can have some side effects — primarily hunger.

The Reason of the Sirtfood Diet

The fundamental reason of the Sirtfood Diet is that sure nourishments, named "sirtfoods," can basically imitate the demonstrated advantages of caloric limitation and fasting by method for actuating sirtuins—proteins in the body (extending from SIRT1 to SIRT7) that control natural pathways, turn certain qualities on and off, and help shield cells from age-related decay

Actuation of SIRT1, for instance, has been appeared in some lab and creature concentrates on instigating the development of new mitochondria, expanding life range, and improve oxidative digestion, which may bolster weight loss and support.

Since fasting and extreme caloric limitation is extremely hard (and often, not fitting), Goggins and Matten built up their dietary arrangement—concentrated on eating heaps of "sirtfoods"— as a more straightforward method to animate the body's sirtuin qualities (in some cases alluded to as "thin qualities") and in this manner increase weight loss and advance by and broad wellbeing.

What makes something a "sirtfood"?

The issue, notwithstanding, is that these nourishments may not contain adequate degrees of these polyphenols to initiate sirtuins in any critical manner. A considerable lot of the examinations connecting polyphenol mixes to expanded sirtuin movement have just been done on profoundly thought types of these mixes.

Now, this all may sound too good to be correct at this point. How is it potentially possible that you can do all of that just with the use of the Sirtfood diet? How can you ever hope to change how your body will respond to the calorie restrictions? If, most of the time, fasting and calorie restriction impact the metabolism, how is it that sirtfoods would not?

These are all fundamental questions to keep in mind. If you are looking at doing something to your body, such as restricting calories, you are absolutely in the right, asking questions about how what you are doing will work and impact your body. Rest assured—your questions will be answered.

Here, we are going to answer four key questions. What are sirtuins? How do sirtuins work for the body? How does calorie restriction impact the body? What are the effects of eating sirtuin-rich foods? As you read, hopefully, you will get an idea of what it is that you can come to expect if you decide that this is the diet for you.

Chapter 2

What are Sirtuins?

Sirtuins are the name for a whole host of proteins that are there to regulate the health of your cells. They help your body to maintain cellular homeostasis, which is a fancy way of saying that they keep the cells balanced to the specifications that they are supposed to be. Homeostasis is found when your body has functions that keep it in the same condition constantly, which is why your body is usually always at right around 98.6 degrees Fahrenheit—that is a way that your body maintains homeostasis. Likewise, your cells have a process to keep them in homeostasis as well—the sirtuins.

Proteins in your body are the workers. Mostly, they work to serve particular roles to keep your body functioning. Think of your body as one big corporation. Within your body, you have different sorts of parts; there are the organs, which serve sort of like the management of a corporation. You have nerves, which connect everything like a network of computers. You have proteins—these are like individual departments within your particular corporation.

Think about it—a corporation will have customer service, human resources, and all sorts of other departments within it so that it can function correctly. They are all departments— but they are each responsible for a different role. Proteins in the body are similar; they are like the departments that keep everything going.

When you take a look at sirtuins, you are looking at a department of proteins that is capable of providing your cells with a way that it can keep the body functioning. In terms of the Sirtfood Diet, they are recognized as the parts that can activate the "skinny gene"—they tell your body to let go of the fats.

How do Sirtuins Work?

You have seven sirtuins in your body—three of them are designed to work in the mitochondria, three of them work in the nucleus, where your DNA is stored so that cells can be run and regulated, and one more is kept in the cytoplasm. They all work together and have very different roles, but they all do one thing: remove acetyl groups from proteins.

Acetyl groups can alter and control the reactions that a cell as—they are like barcodes on proteins that tell other proteins what they are and how to interact with them. Through the process of deacetylation, sirtuins work to recognize that a molecule in the body has an acetyl group, and they then move it, allowing the molecule to get ready to do its job. Necessarily, the sirtuins are able to get everything ready to work.

In terms of the Sirtfood Diet, then you can expect that the act of fasting and restricting calories will change the way that the body is working. It will then allow for the sirtuins throughout the body to have an effect on how it works. Fat synthesis is repressed. The body is told not to uptake the cholesterol.

The body can reject the fatty acids. Because fasting will up the level of activation of sirtuins, it allows for fats to not be stored. They are activated for use instead, allowing the body to burn them for energy when it is needed.

The barcodes for those acetyl groups on the fats in the body mainly get scanned, and the sirtuins tell the molecule to get ready for work—which in this case, will be making use of the way that the body processes it. The fat goes through oxidation, gets used up, and therefore is lost from the body.

What Happens When I Restrict Calories?

When you restrict calories, you necessarily tell your body that food is not available to it. You have a healthy metabolism that is meant to tell you when to eat to make sure that you continuously have energy.

Think of hunger like that little gas light coming on in your car—it is there to remind you that you are running low on stored gas and that filling it up soon would probably be a good idea. Your hunger is there to keep you topped off mostly—it does not want you to drop below a certain level. However, when you restrict your calories, you do not provide that extra food.
This means that your body has to shift gears—it can no longer count on being topped off to provide the energy levels that are needed, and the deficit is created.

When that happens, the body has a tremendous back-up mechanism that your car does not. Your body has stores of fat that can be broken down when there is a deficit in calories. When your body cannot get what it requires, it is able to work instead to get those calories elsewhere; it can provide itself with energy by breaking down that fat.

Does that sound familiar? It is quite like the function of the sirtuins! Permanently, due to the threat to homeostasis in the body, the sirtuins activate and inhibit insulin while encouraging the oxidation of the fat in the body.

Usually, during calorie restriction, there are also other side effects, such as losing muscle, but that will be able to be protected against in different ways. During mild to moderate calorie restriction, weight loss is average and expected without too many other issues. One of the more common ways of creating a deficit in calories is through the use of exercising while also restricting calories.

What Happens When I Eat Sirtuin-Rich Food?

When you eat sirtuin-rich foods, you are bringing more of those sirtuins into your body and therefore have more access to them for breaking down and using. This is highly beneficial to you—you will have them readily available in your body to be able to use them.

Even more beneficial, however, is the fact that so many of the foods that are rich in sirtuin are typically also highly healthy for you. You are looking to consume primarily all sorts of fruits and vegetables that will help you to keep your body happy, healthy, and ready to tackle the world.

Sirtfoods are a newfound gathering of nourishments that turn on a ground-breaking recycling activity in the body that leaches out cell waste and remove fat. They do this by initiating our sirtuin 'thin' qualities – similar qualities enacted by exercise and fasting.

Alongside fat consuming, Sirtfoods likewise have the extraordinary capacity to satisfy craving and increment muscle work usually. It is settled that the way of life eating the most Sirtfoods has been the least fatty and most advantageous on the planet.

Sirtuin rich foods are typically foods dubbed "superfoods"—those that are full of all sorts of what your body needs to survive and thrive. The increased nutrient content in these foods on their own is already a compelling reason to add them into your diet—the addition of the sirtuins is just icing on top.

Remember, the Sirtfood Diet is all about healthy eating—it is meant to keep your body healthy with the rapid weight loss being secondary to it.

Chapter 3

The Pros and Cons of Sirt Food Diet

For every diet, eating plan, and lifestyle, there are both pros and cons. For one person, a diet might not work because of health restrictions, whereas for another person, it may be the ideal fit.

You can only decide if the Sirt diet is the correct fit for you by understanding both the pros and cons. Try discussing these with your doctor, and you can work together to help you enjoy a healthy, balanced, and successful Sirt diet.

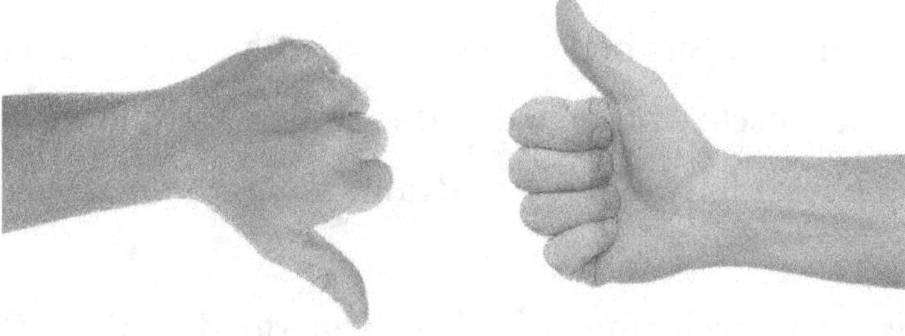

The Pros of Sirt Food Diet

- Pro: Great Weight Loss

Losing weight is hard. But it doesn't have to be. With the Sirt diet, you are able to have a manageable plan, delicious food, steady weight loss, and weight maintenance. People regularly lose five to seven pounds on the plan, and this is only during a single round of both phases.

If you repeatedly practice the first phase every three to four months, you could be losing weight steadily every month. Because of this, you can lose, however, much weight you need on the Sirt diet, as long as you put in the time and effort. Whether you only want to lose five pounds or want to lose a hundred, you can steadily progress toward your goal.

- Pro: Produced the Same Results as Fasting and Exercise

Exercise and fasting create a cellular metabolic response that causes accelerated fat loss in a way that diet alone generally cannot. However, the Sirt diet is also able to tune-into this weight loss caused by what is fondly called the 'skinny gene' by implementing Sirtfoods and calorie restriction. This is all possible because Sirtfoods contain polyphenols, a plant compound that reactors the same at biological sirtuins.

Because of this, sirtuins are able to react with the body's sirtuin receptors, triggering fat loss more quickly than would otherwise be possible. As this is paired with calorie restriction, it can boost the effects even further.

- Pro: Sustained Weight Loss, when the Lifestyle is Sustained

There are many diets that once you stop, the weight comes right back. But who wants to have their weight yo-yo every year? Who wants to spend the time, energy, and effort losing weight, only for all of it to come right back? Who has room in their closet for clothes of three different sizes?

Thankfully, the Sirt diet is not only a weight loss diet but also a maintenance lifestyle. Once you reach your goal weight, you can then maintain it by simply enjoying your daily balanced meals full of Sirt foods and a serving of green juice.

You can still enjoy your favorite foods, even pizza. Still, by regularly incorporating Sirtfoods into your diet and eating your doctor's caloric recommendation for you, then you can maintain weight naturally and easily.

- Pro: Eat Healthy, Balanced, and Delicious Meals

There are many diets out there that simply allow you to eat a bunch of breakfast cereal, frozen meals, nothing but juice, or just salads. The Sirtfood Diet isn't like this. Sure, you'll drink some green juice, but you aren't drinking this in place of meals, but rather alongside them.

You can regularly eat salads, as they are natural and healthy. But, if you don't like salads, then you don't have to include them. There are other ways to eat healthfully and incorporate vegetables than eating a cold salad for lunch.

You also don't have to stick with bland cereals or frozen meals. Instead, you can create a variety of recipes fitted to your taste buds and lifestyle, whether you enjoy Italian pizza, Indian curry, or traditional American fare. It doesn't matter.

You can incorporate the types of meals you enjoy as part of your daily life. This will give you food that is not only healthy, balanced, and delicious, but that also fits your lifestyle.

- Pro: It is Simple to Follow

Many diets are complicated. They require you to not only count calories, but also fats, carbohydrates, and fiber. They may require you to keep to a strict schedule. The Sirt diet isn't like that.

All you have to do is follow the recommended calorie consumption for a given phrase while enjoying plenty of Sirtfoods. That's it. It's that easy. But this becomes even easier in the second phase and during maintenance, because you can be more forgiving of calories at these times, allowing you to take it easy while losing or maintaining weight.

- Pro: Cooking Right for You

Some people love to be in the kitchen, whereas others have little time or energy for it. Whichever type of person you are, you can find a fit on the Sirt diet. There are many delicious recipes that you can use, or you could even customize old family favorite recipes to give them a Sirtfood twist.

But, if you have little time to be in the kitchen, there are also more accessible options. Many people will simply prepare salads ahead of time at the beginning of the week and store them in the fridge until mealtime.

Along with this, many people will simply roast a chicken or two, a couple of pans of Sirtfood vegetables, and make a pot of buckwheat on the stove. By storing these simple meal components in the fridge or freezer at all times, a person can simply grab one component of each for a delicious and healthy meal. Alternate what seasoning you add or create sauces for more diversity.

- Pro: Sirtfoods is Good for You

The human body is full of free radicals, which create cellular DNA damage and accelerate aging and promote disease. This is why many health products are specifically meant to reduce free radical damage.

Sirtfoods can naturally reduce the free radicals in your body, thus slowing down the speed of aging and disease. This is because Sirtfoods contain many potent compounds that not only fight against the free radicals but actively work to protect your cellular DNA.

Of course, there is no way to stop aging. But, Sirtfoods can promote less rapid and healthier aging, so that you can enjoy your old age to the fullest.

- Pro: You Can Enjoy Wine and Dark Chocolate

Lastly, we all have our favorite foods. Some of the peoples' most common favorite foods are chocolate and wine, both of which are great Sirtfoods! Of course, this doesn't mean you can eat these foods without limit, but in moderation, they can be a great addition to your Sirtfood diet.

When eating chocolate, try to look for darker chocolate with less sugar. Ideally, you will buy chocolate, which is 70% dark or more. Cocoa powder is a great option, as it is pure chocolate without added sugars or fat.

You can easily make delicious chocolaty Sirtfood desserts with cocoa, without relying on a manufacturer to not add unnecessarily high amounts of unhealthy ingredients. For instance, you will find a delicious recipe for chocolate ice cream, which is much healthier than anything you could find in the store.

You should also be careful with red wine. It is not recommended during the first phase, but rather for the second phase and maintenance. This is because, during the first phase, your calories are minimal. Because of this, all that you consume needs to prioritize, giving your body the nutrients it needs to get through the day.

While red wine is a Sirtfood, it offers little to maintain your body's function. Alcohol in excess can limit the metabolism and weight loss. To avoid this, you shouldn't drink more than the recommended servings for your weight and body type. It is also important to remember that because your calories are restricted in the first phase, if you did drink alcohol, it could cause you to get drunk easily and have more severe hangovers.

While you should always be careful about not enjoying anything in excess, this is especially the case with alcohol and sweets. Thankfully, it is easy to enjoy them in moderation to improve your Sirt diet and your enjoyment of the process.

The Cons of Sirt Food Diet

- Con: Individuals can Restrict Protein and Lose muscle

On the Sirt diet, most people can maintain muscle or even gain muscle while losing weight! However, it is always possible for individual people to make mistakes, especially if they are busy, tired, or mistaken about how the diet works. In this case, many people may not include enough protein in their daily lives to maintain muscle mass.

While this is not usually a problem when it does occur, a person can feel defeated and confused as to why it happened. The truth is, while many people only think of the Sirtfoods when they are on the Sirt diet, other sources of nutrition are just as important.

You shouldn't forsake protein just to reduce your calorie count further or increase your Sirtfood consumption. Both protein and Sirtfoods are essential and should be treated as such. If you eat plenty of protein on the Sirt diet, then you generally won't have a problem, just like on any other diet.

- Con: It is Possible to Over Limit Calories

Eating 1,000 calories a day for three days is a significant calorie reduction. But that isn't to say it isn't possible. Some people may be able to restrict their calories to such a degree, while others may not. That is okay.

Some may find that the calorie restriction is too much for your health and lifestyle than you can simply take it slowly by increasing your calorie consumption slightly.

This will slow your weight loss, but it will also reduce any side effects caused by calorie reduction such as hunger and fatigue.

- Con: It is Not Recommended for Everyone

While the Sirt diet is generally safe, it is not recommended for everyone. Most notably, people who are pregnant, breastfeeding, underweight, and children should not practice the first phase. Similarly, people with certain illnesses or disabilities might not be able to practice the first phase.

But this does not mean the second phase is inaccessible. Most people who are unable to practice the first phase are still able to practice the second phase, allowing them to experience the positives of the diet with fewer of the drawbacks.

- Con: Hunger Cravings

Hunger cravings and pangs can be severe; I won't lie. This is one of the most difficult aspects of dieting for many people. But it is often a natural course when you change how you eat, no matter the diet.

The intensity of your cravings will differ from person to person. While some people only experience slight cravings for the first three days, others might have a more difficult adjustment period.

The good news is that there are ways you can lessen cravings. I recommend eating most of your food during the first three days of the first phase in the evening. This will allow you to go to bed full, so that hunger won't keep you awake. You are also less likely to make mistakes when tired this way.

Con: Few Studies on the Sirt Diet

While there is much known on Sirtfoods, weight loss, dieting, and exercise, the Sirt diet itself is relatively new.

Because of this, while we might have a lot of general studies that can give us a picture of the effects of the diet, few complete studies are specifically researching the Sirt diet itself.

Chapter 4

Sirt Food and its Relationship to Building Muscle and Anti-Aging

Muscle Building

Sirtuins are a group of proteins with different effects. Sirt-1 is the protein responsible for causing the body to burn fat rather than muscle for energy, which is a miracle for weight loss. Another useful aspect of Sirt-1 is its ability to improve skeletal muscle.

Skeletal muscle is all the muscles you voluntarily control, such as the muscles in your limbs, back, shoulders, and so on. There are two other types, and cardiac muscle is what the heart is formed of, while the smooth muscle is your involuntary muscles – which includes muscles around your blood vessels, face, and various parts of organs and other tissues.

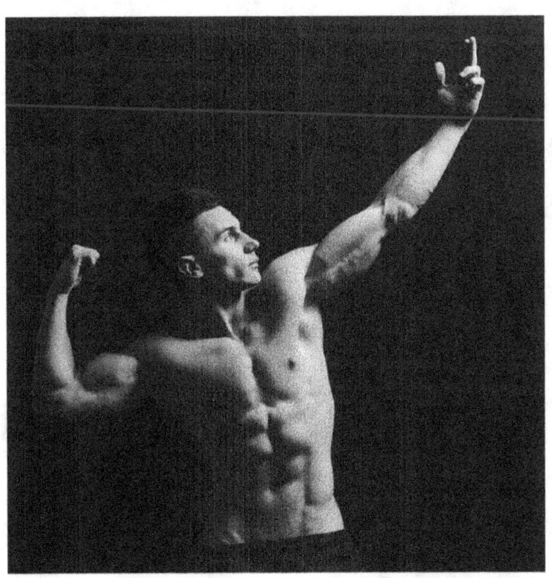

Skeletal muscle is separated into two different groups, the blandly named type-1 and type-2. Type 1 muscle is effective at continued, sustained activity, whereas type-2 muscle is effective at short, intense periods of activity. So, for example, you would predominantly use type-1 muscles for jogging, but type-2 muscles for sprinting.

Sirt-1 protects the type-1 muscles, but not the type-2 muscle, which is still broken down for energy. Therefore, holistic muscle mass drops when fasting, even though type-1 skeletal muscle mass increases.

Sirt-1 also influences how the muscles work. Sirt-1 is produced by the muscle cells, but the ability to produce Sirt-1 decreases as the muscle ages. As a result, muscle is harder to build as you age and doesn't grow as fast in response to exercise. A lack of sirt-1 also causes the muscles to become tired quicker and gradually decline over time.

When you start to consider these effects of Sirt-1, you can start to form a picture of why fasting helps keep the body supple. Fasting releases Sirt-1, which in turn helps skeletal muscle grow and stay in good shape. Sirt-1 is also released by consuming sirtuin activators, giving the sirtfood diet its muscle retaining power.

Why Maintain Good Muscles?

Maybe you're asking what the deal is? Primarily, you will look so much better. Shedding off fat, but being able to retain muscle, will lead to your aspired toned, athletic and lean physique. But more importantly, again, you'll stay looking good.

The Skeletal muscle is the main factor that is responsible for our body's energy expenditure every day. What I mean is the more muscle you fain, the more energy you can utilize, even when you are stationary. This will aid in supporting further loss of weight and will increase the success rate, long-term.

With the usual dieting, loss of weight will come from both muscle and fat loss, and with that, we can observe metabolic rate that is declining. The result of that will make the body regain weight when past eating habits are resumed. But through maintaining muscle mass with the consumption of Sirtfoods, you will be burning more fat with a lesser drop-in metabolic rate. This is the perfect start and foundation for successful long-term weight loss.

Besides, muscle mass and role are a variable of healthy aging and well-being, and maintaining muscle hinders the production of chronic diseases like osteoporosis, diabetes, keeping us mobile into older age too. Another important effect is it will keep us happy, sirtuins have benefits over stress-related disorders, including reduction of depression.

In total, loss of weight while protecting the muscle is a big factor and will always give us beneficial outcomes. This is one unique feature of The Sirtfood Diet.

Sirtfood vs. Fasting

This leads us into a great question: if sirtuin stimulation increases muscle growth, then why can we lose muscle if we quickly? In the end, fasting triggers our sirtuin genes too. And herein lies one of those significant downsides of fasting.

Bear with us while we delve deeper into just how this works. Not all of the skeletal muscle is made equal. We now have two major forms, conveniently referred to as type-1, along with type-2.

Type-1 muscle can be utilized for longer-duration actions, whereas type-2 muscle can be used for small bursts of intense action. And here is where it becomes fascinating: fasting raises SIRT1 activity just in type-1 muscle fibers, maybe not in type-2.[7] Thus type-1 muscle fiber dimension is preserved and even markedly increases if we quickly.[8] Regrettably, in total contrast to what occurs in type-1 fibers through fasting, SIRT1 quickly declines in type-2 fibers.

This implies fat-burning melts, and rather muscle begins to divide to give fuel. Thus, fasting is also a double-edged sword for joints, together with our type-2 fibers carrying a bang. Type-2 fibers are that which contain the majority of our muscle building definition. Therefore, even when our type-1 fiber mass raises, we see a generally significant reduction of muscle together with fasting.

If we can halt the breakdown, then it might not just make us look great visually but also help encourage additional fat reduction. And the means to do so is to fight the fall in SIRT1 at type-2 muscle fiber caused by fasting. Within an elegant mice research, scientists at Harvard Medical School place this on the evaluation, also demonstrated by arousing SIRT1 action in type-2 fibers through fasting, the signs for muscle dysfunction were changed, and muscle weight loss did not happen. The researchers moved one step farther and analyzed the effects of greater SIRT1 action on muscle once the mice were fed instead of regretting and found that it triggered quite rapid muscle development. Within only a week, muscle fibers with high degrees of SIRT1 activity revealed an astonishing 20 percent boost in fat.

These findings are extremely much like the results of the Sirtfood Diet trial, even though our analysis was significantly milder in effect. By upping SIRT1 action through ingesting a diet rich in Sirtfoods, nearly all participants had no muscle loss --and for most, using it just being a medium quick, muscle mass improved.

Anti-aging and Cell Repair

We're done talking about muscle mass, but now let's look at another relationship, sirtuins and cell repair. The great effects of SIRT1 on muscle expand to its functionality too. As muscle undergoes aging, its capacity to activate SIRT1 lessens. In effect, it will lessen its responsiveness to the positive benefits of exercise. It will lead to the great possibility of damage from free radicals and inflammation, which will result in oxidative stress. Muscles slowly get weaker, wither, and get tired easily.

But if we make the activation of SIRT1 higher, we can stop the age-related decline. Sirtuin is known as the natural regulator of the cell metabolic activity; From the repair of the DNA to the synthesis of proteins, the Sirtuins play their part in every cellular activity which leads to increased metabolic activity. In simple words, the Sirtuin- rich food can help boost the working speed of the body and enables it to burn all the calories quickly.

Truly, by the activation of SIRT1 to hinder the loss of muscle function and mass we usually see with aging, we observe a lot of related health benefits, which include stopping loss of bone mass, preventing inflammaging, mobility improvements, and better quality of life.

Sirtuins have a profound impact on the cell cycle. With age, the cell loses its ability to quickly, repair, heal, or reproduce itself. Sirtuins can ensure all these processes. With the sirtuins rich food, a person can not only look young, but he can also feel young on the inside. Besides these known advantages, a sirtfood diet can also prevent inflammation and reduce its stress.

Chapter 5

Sirt Food and its Relationship to Weight Loss

Weight loss

Weight loss, being the obvious benefit of this diet, is most sought for by the dieters. The first phase of the sirtfood diet works most for this cause; during this phase, a person not only consumes Sirtuin rich food but also cuts his caloric intake down 1000-1500 calories per day. Moreover, the good use of green juices and Sirtuin food, together with all these measures, can help the body to metabolize the excess fats and lose about 2-3 pounds quickly.

All sirtuins, including SIRT1 important for sensing energy status and in protection against metabolic stress. They coordinate cellular response towards Caloric Restriction (CR) in an organism. SIRT1 diverse location and allows cells to easily sense changes in the level of energy anywhere in the mitochondria, nucleus, and cytoplasm.

It is associated with metabolic health through deacetylation of several target proteins such as muscles, liver, endothelium, heart, and adipose tissue.

Sirtuins, Fasting and Metabolic Activities

SIRT1, SIRT6, and SIRT7 are localized in the nucleus where they take part in the deacetylation of customers to influence gene expression epigenetically. SIRT2 is located in the cytosol, while SIRT3, SIRT4, and SIRT5 are located in the mitochondria where they regulate metabolic enzyme activities as well as moderate oxidative stress.

SIRT1, as most studies with regards to metabolism, aid in mediating the physiological adaptation to diets. Several studies have shown the impact of sirtuins on Caloric Restriction. Sirtuins deacetylase non-histone proteins that define pathways involved during the metabolic adaptation when there are metabolic restrictions. Caloric Restriction, on the other hand, causes the induction of expression of SIRT1 in humans. Mutations that lead to loss of function in some sirtuins genes can lead to a reduction in the outputs of caloric restrictions. Therefore, sirtuins have the following metabolic functions:

The Liver regulates the body glucose homeostasis. During fasting or caloric restriction, glucose level becomes low, resulting in a sudden shift in hepatic metabolism to glycogen breakdown and then to gluconeogenesis to maintain glucose supply as well as ketone body production to mediate the deficit in energy.

Also, during caloric restriction or fasting, there is muscle activation and liver oxidation of fatty acids produced during lipolysis in white adipose tissue. For this switch to occur, there are several transcription factors involved to adapt to energy deprivation. SIRT1 intervenes during the metabolic switch to see the energy deficit.

At the initial stage of the fasting that is the post glycogen breakdown phase, there is the production of glucagon by the pancreatic alpha cells to active gluconeogenesis in the Liver through the cyclic amp response element-binding protein (CREB). CREB regulated transcription coactivator 2 (CRTC2), the coactivator.

Is the fasting gets prolonged, the effect is canceled out and is being replaced by SIRT1 mediated CRTC2 deacetylase resulting in targeting of the coactivator for ubiquitin/ proteasome-mediated destruction? SIRT1, on the other hand, initiates the next stage of gluconeogenesis through acetylation and activation of peroxisome proliferator-activated receptor coactivator one alpha, which is the coactivator necessary for forkhead box O1.

In addition to the ability of SIRT1 to support gluconeogenesis, coactivator one alpha is required during the mitochondrial biogenesis necessary for the liver to accommodate the reduction in energy status. SIRT1 also activates fatty acid oxidation through deacetylation and activation of the nuclear receptor to increase energy production. SIRT1, when involved in acetylation and repression of glycolytic enzymes such as phosphoglycerate mutate 1, can lead to shutting down of the production of energy through glycolysis.

SIRT6, on the other hand, can be served as a co-repressor for hypoxia-inducible Factor 1 Alpha to repress glycolysis. Since SIRT6 can transcriptionally be induced by SIRT1, sirtuins can coordinate the duration of time for each fasting phase.

Aside from glucose homeostasis, the liver also overtakes in lipid and cholesterol homeostasis during fasting. When there are caloric restrictions, the synthesis of fat and cholesterol in the liver is turned off, while lipolysis in the white adipose tissue commences. The SIRT1, upon fasting, causes acetylation of steroid regulatory element-binding protein (SREBP) and targets the protein to destroy the ubiquitin-professor system.

The result is that fat cholesterol synthesis will repress. During the regulation of cholesterol homeostasis, SIRT1 regulates the oxysterol receptor, thereby assisting the reversal of cholesterol transport from peripheral tissue through upregulation of the oxysterol receptor target gene ATP-binding cassette transporter A1 (ABCA1).

Further modulation of the cholesterol regulatory loop can be achieved via bile acid receptor, that's necessary for the biosynthesis of cholesterol catabolic and bile acid pathways. SIRT6 also participates in the regulation of cholesterol levels by repressing the expression and post-translational cleavage of SREBP1/2, into the active form. Furthermore, in the circadian regulation of metabolism, SIRT1 participates through the regulation of cell circadian clock.

Mitochondrial SIRT3 is crucial in the oxidation of fatty acid in mitochondria. Fasting or caloric restrictions can result in the up-regulation of activities and levels of SIRT3 to aid fatty acid oxidation through deacetylation of long-chain specific acyl-CoA dehydrogenase. SIRT3 can also cause activation of ketogenesis and the urea cycle in the liver.

SIRT1 also Add it in the metabolic regulation in the muscle and white adipose tissue. Fasting causes an increase in the level of SIRT1, leading to deacetylation of coactivator one alpha, which in turn causes genes responsible for fat oxidation to get activated.

The reduction in energy level also activates AMPK, which will activate the expression of coactivator one alpha. The combined effects of the two processes will give rise to increased mitochondrial biogenesis together with fatty acid oxidation in the muscle.

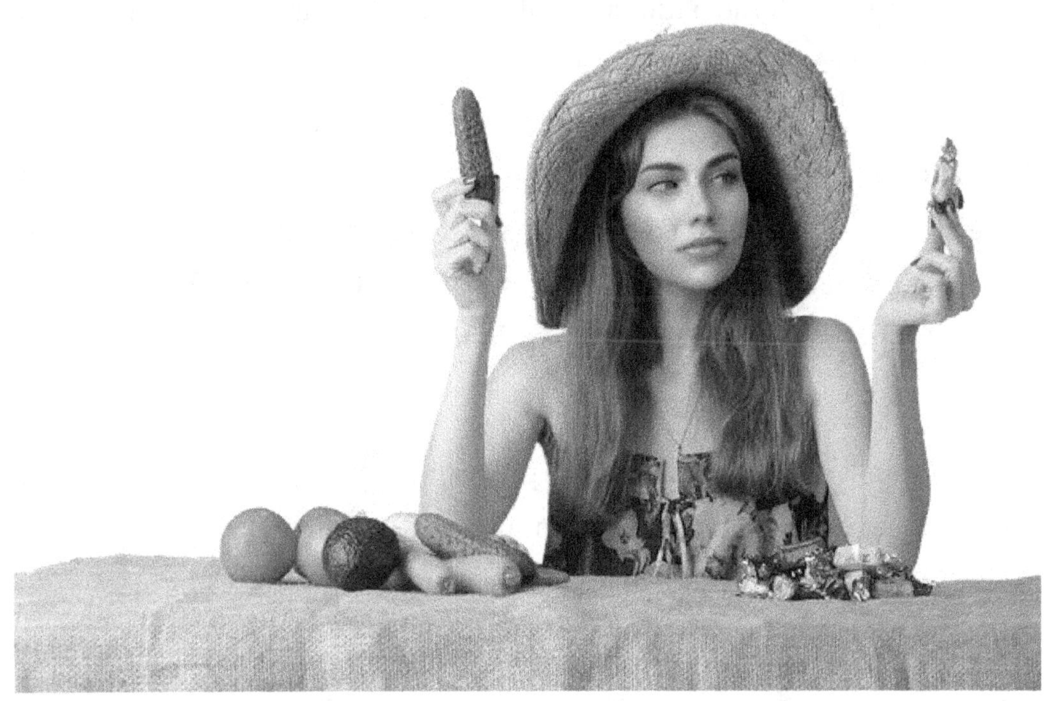

Chapter 6

Sirtfood Diet and Ways to Make it Efficient

The plan asserts that eating particular foods can trigger your "lean receptor" pathway and possess you losing seven pounds in 7 days. Foods such as ginseng, dark chocolate, and milk contain a natural compound called polyphenols, which mimic the results of fasting and exercise. Strawberries, red onions, cinnamon, and garlic will also be powerful Sirtfoods.

These foods can activate the sirtuin pathway to help activate weight reduction. The science seems appealing. However, in reality, there is very little research to back up these claims. Plus, the guaranteed speed of weight reduction from the very first week is quite quick and perhaps not in accord with the national institute of health safe fat loss recommendations of a couple of pounds each week.

The diet includes 2 stages:

- Stage 1 endure for 2 days. For the initial 3 days, you will be drinking three glasses of sirtfood green juice along with something meal full of Sirtfoods for an overall total of 1000 calories. From days 4 to 7, you will just drink two juices and 2 meals for a total of 1,500 calories.

- Stage 2 is really a 14day maintenance program, though it's created to your shed weight steadily (perhaps not maintain your present weight). Daily is composed of three balanced Sirtfood meals plus also one green juice.

Later those 3 weeks, you are invited to keep on eating a diet full of Sirtfoods and drinking with a green juice each day. It's possible to discover several Sirtfood cookbooks on the web and also recipes to the Sirtfood internet site. 1 green juice recipe entirely on the Sirtfood internet site is made up of a combination of spinach and other leafy greens Matcha, ginger celery, carrot, green apple and, lemon juice. Lovage and Buckwheat may also be things that can be advocated for use on your green juice. The diet urges that juices need to be drawn up in a juicer, so perhaps not really a blender, so that it tastes better. Below are tips on how to make most of your diet plan

Protein Power

Aside from the greens we consume into our Sirtfood Diet, we must practice eating Sirtfood meals rich in protein to reap maximum benefits. Leucine, a building block of dietary protein, shows to have added benefits in the stimulation of SIRT1 to increase fat burning and improvement in blood sugar.

Apart from that, leucine plays one more role, and this is where its symbiotic connection with Sirtfoods truly prospers. It has a potent ability to stimulate anabolism (building) in our cells, muscle in particular, which needs tons of energy, and in turn, our mitochondria (energy factories) have to work more.

This results in a need in our cells for the activity of Sirtfoods. You can remember, one effect of Sirtfood is the stimulation of mitochondria to be made, improvement of their efficiency, and let them burn fat. Therefore, our bodies require them to meet his added demand for energy. The consequence is that by joining Sirtfoods with dietary protein, we can observe a harmonious effect that will boost activation of sirtuin and, in the end, will get you to burn fat to fuel muscle growth and better health. This is the reason why the inclusion of protein in meals is essential.

Fish rich in oil are good choices for protein to supplement the effect of Sirtfoods since it is rich in omega-3 fatty acids in addition to their protein content. It is a well-known fact about the health benefits one can gain from omega 3 fish oils, and now studies show that these benefits will be enhanced in the sirtuin genes.

Eating Early

When it comes to our eating habits, the philosophy you must embrace is "the earlier, the better, "where we do not eat beyond 7 p.m. Why? The first reason is to obtain the natural satiating effect of Sirtfoods. There are more good effects on consuming a meal that will keep one full, energized, and satisfied as you go about your day than consuming time feeling hunger only to consume and stay full as you take your sleep through the night.

The second most important reason, which is to retain habits of eating in line with your internal body clock. All people have a built-in body clock known as a circadian rhythm that modulates a lot of our body functions in accordance with the time of the day, and it also has an influence on how our body manages the food we intake.

Our body clocks work in coordination, following the hints of the light-dark cycle of the sun. WE are naturally made to be active during the daytime and less active during the night. Therefore, our body readies us up in handing food most effectively during the daytime, when we are expected to be active, and there's the presence of light and less effective during night time, where we are expected to sleep and rest.

To one degree, we can train our body clocks to be in sync with various schedules, like evening chronotypes, who like to or most prone to eat and be active later in the day. But not being able to do so, people will have increased vulnerability to muscle loss, fat gain and metabolic problems, and of course, lack of good sleep. This is why we see those working night shifts tend to have higher rates of metabolic diseases and higher rates of obesity due to their unusual sleeping patterns.

One good news is that consuming sirtuin foods plays an important role in the synchronization of our body clock. The truth is, several types of research have proven that polyphenols found in Sirtfoods can modulate body clocks and can adjust circadian rhythms positively.

This means, if a person cannot prevent eating beyond 7 pm, eating Sirtfoods with your meals will be able t lessen the bad effects. Truly, one of the continual bits of feedback people hear from those doing Sirtfood Diet is just their sleep quality improved well, suggesting great effects on synchronizing circadian rhythm.

Focus on Taste

A basic problem with traditional dieting is that it usually makes for a bad dining experience. It hinders us from experiencing the pleasure of eating tasty foods, which leaves us the feeling of dissatisfaction. It is important to retain the joy of food while trying to maintain a healthy weight. That is why it is with great delight to know that Sirtfoods works in satisfying our desire for taste. It's a win-win situation: Sirtfoods tastes greats and helps us boost our health.

Let's study more on how this function. The taste receptors dictate how tasty our food is and how satisfied we can get from consuming it. It can happen with the 7 main Taste receptors, which are certainly present in sirtfoods. The following are the seven main taste receptors and sirtuin food examples that you can eat.

- sweet (strawberries, dates)

- salty (celery, fish)

- sour (strawberries)

- bitter (cocoa, kale, endive, extra virgin olive oil, green tea)

- pungent (chilies, garlic, extra virgin olive oil)

- astringent (green tea, red wine)

- umami (soy, fish, meat)

Crucially, what we have discovered is that the greater the sirtuin-activating properties of food, the more powerfully it stimulates those taste centers, and the more gratification we get from the food we eat. Importantly, it also means that we satisfy our appetite quicker, and our desire to eat more is reduced accordingly.

This is a key reason why those who follow a Sirtfood-rich diet are pleasantly fuller more quickly.

Chapter 7

The Best Sirt Foods

The principle is simple: bet everything on "superfoods," such as apples, onions, green tea ... or dark chocolate and red wine. These are natural activators of the sirtuin enzymes present in our body and themselves endowed with the capacity to stimulate the "discomfort of thinness."

The sirtfood diet is based on the principle that consuming foods rich in sirtuins is enough to lose weight without actually having to deprive yourself. Sirtuins are proteins naturally synthesized by the body, which increase the body's ability to burn fat, activate the metabolism, and consolidate muscle mass. They also have an anti-aging effect.

With the Sirt food Diet, you don't have to pay attention to the contents of your basket or deprive yourself of delicious chocolate desserts to keep your figure. The principle of this slimming diet is simple: consume foods rich in sirtuins. Sirtuins are fat-burning enzymes that activate metabolism and help consolidate muscle mass.

Because of their richness in sirtuins, these foods, called superfoods, lead to rapid weight loss by removing excess fat, improve muscle performance, and keep you on track for your health. Favoring them in your diet is, therefore, an effective way to shed those extra pounds and reshape your figure.

According to its two founders, the Sirt Food Diet would have the same effects as a sports activity, that is to say, that it would burn the maximum amount of fat and strengthen physical health through the consumption of these superfoods.

While it may not be a healthy diet, there are many great purposes why most important Sirt foods are in a weight loss plan, including berries, kale, ginger, green tea, olive oil, and turmeric. Here is an introduction to some of the most-rich and recommended Sirt foods - only enjoy them as part of a healthy diet with various choices of other healthy foods.

1. Chia seeds

In the world of Sirt foods, chia seeds are considered to be moderately sirtuin inactivating foods, which the authors of the Sirt food diet describe in their book as the equivalent of walking and getting into a food intensive sweating session in the gym.

Whether the claims contain water or not, there is no debate that chia seeds pack an incredible amount of nutrients in a small package, making them an efficient way to boost nutrient deficiencies like fiber (11 grams per ounce, or 44 percent of the daily value) and heart-healthy omega-3 fats (five grams per ounce). Chia is also a good source of vegetable protein. Simply sprinkle over a smoothie bowl, add to the smoothies or mix with oatmeal.

2. Cinnamon

In a study presented at the 2017 American Society for Biochemistry and Molecular Biology's annual meeting, researchers used a computer model to determine whether cinnamon activated Sirt-1 and found promising compounds. This is not proof yet, but an interesting building block for future research.

But cinnamon is still on the list of Sirt foods because it contains strong polyphenols, herbal compounds with antioxidant and anti-inflammatory properties. And studies are suggesting that cinnamon can aid in controlling blood sugar by making digestions of carb slower and improvement on how the body responds to insulin. It goes well with coffee, hot chocolate, cabbage, roasted pumpkin, soups, smoothies, and spices for lean pork.

3. Cocoa

The suggested nutrient in cocoa that is very potent in activating sirtuin is known as epicatechin. This antioxidant can also be commonly found in tea and grapes. In a 2016 animal study, cocoa increased Sirtuin-1, but keep in mind that the jump from mouse to human is a big one.

As a food rich in polyphenols, pure cocoa promotes healthy blood circulation, which is important for the sup of nutrients and oxygen as well as for general health. Keep in mind that the good effects are yielded from the cacao plant and not from the added salt sugar and fat like what you get from supermarket chocolate bars. Seek for the proportion, highest one, chocolate you can get the greatest benefits.

4. Coffee

Coffee is the primary source of antioxidants in the U.S. diet. His sirt food creed comes from his polyphenol, caffeic acid. Animal studies with caffeic acid (and another antioxidant polyphenol in coffee, chlorogenic acid) showed that obese mice lost weight, including belly fat.

It also lowered insulin, triglyceride, and cholesterol levels while increasing fatty acid oxidation and blocking the formation of new fat cells in the liver. While several tests were done on mice rather than humans, the results yield that the coffee beans have essential components that can greatly aid in improving body weight and how it has a great response in breaking down the body's fats.

5. Olive oil

The suspected sirtuin-activating polyphenols in virgin olive oil are hydroxytyrosol and oleuropein. The known fact by a lot of people is that olive oil is a primary ingredient of the Mediterranean diet, which is heart-friendly and good support in managing weight.

It is rich in monounsaturated fats that improve cholesterol when it replaces saturated fats or refined carbohydrates. Extra virgin varieties have the most complex polyphenol profiles, although they decrease with air, heat, and time. Many bottles have a harvest date so you can find the freshest olive oil.

6. Ginger

Ginger is a cousin of turmeric, which is also on the list of Sirt foods. It contains gingerol, which has anti-inflammatory and antioxidant properties. It has long been used as a natural cure for motion sickness and can generally help with nausea and dizziness.

Fresh chopped ginger gives turkey burgers a high-contrast aroma. It is also a peppery and invigorating addition to smoothies and salad dressings. Fry it with other flavors like onions and garlic before adding vegetables for a quick weekly side dish. (Pro tip: use a spoon and some pressure to peel the gnarled skin slightly.)

7. Matcha

The well-known long-lived, healthy population groups of Japan may like something with their love for tea. Green tea is included as a staple food due to its antioxidant epigallocatechin gallate (EGCG). The authors of the Sirtfood Diet particularly recommend the powdered Matcha green tea form.

Regardless of whether you prefer green, white, oolong, or black, tea drinkers tend to have lower bad LDL cholesterol and better HDL cholesterol. Regular tea also contains some caffeine for an extra boost. Enjoy it in smoothies or as a poaching liquid for cod - or just drink a cup as part of your morning ritual.

8. Raspberries

Raspberries and other berries such as strawberries and blackberries have adopted sirtuin-activating polyphenols. No wonder that berries are antioxidant superstars. Raspberries, especially quercetin and gallic acid, and strawberries are notable sources of fisetin. Fresh summer raspberries are great on their own, and frozen raspberries can be enjoyed all year round in a deserted smoothie or an unexpectedly fresh salsa. Both are high in fiber and vitamin C.

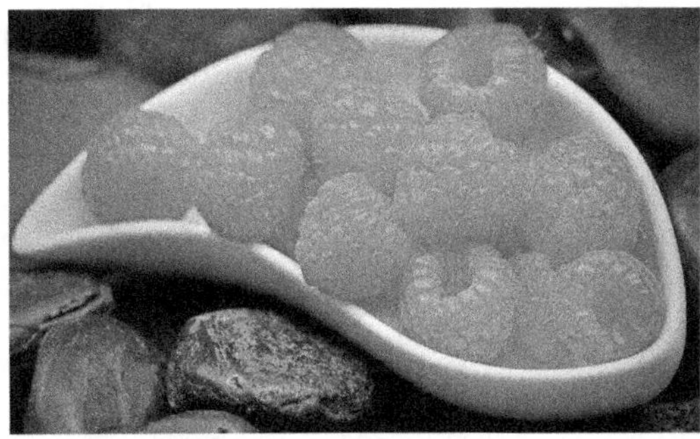

9. Kale

Kohl's most important antioxidants in the Sirt food diet are kaempferol and quercetin, which have been tested primarily in laboratories and animals for their anti-inflammatory effects. They are undoubtedly waging a radical struggle on your behalf.

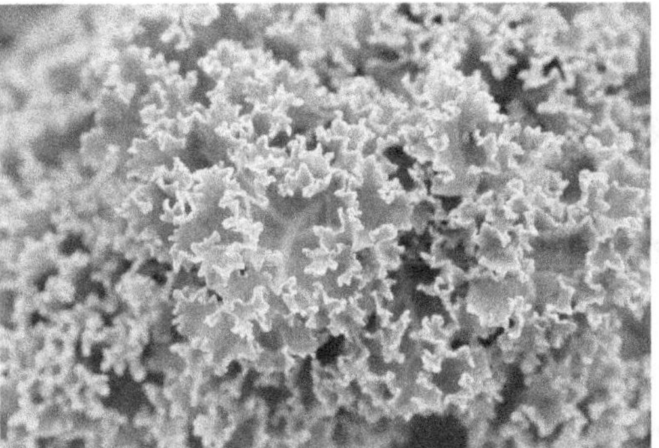

And as if that wasn't enough, a cup of kale contains twice as much vitamin A and more vitamin C than an orange. Remove the stems, roll them, and cut them crosswise into tiny slanted strands (chiffonade) before combining them with your preferred dressing for a few minutes. Put this kale strand that has been marinated and the fruits you have nearby to your grain like wheat berry, farro, freekeh, or sorghum for an easy and nutritious whole grain salad.

10. Red wine

Red wine has made a name for itself in health circles because it contains resveratrol, a polyphenol that can activate sirtuins. Human observational studies suggest that moderate intake could have health benefits for older adults, especially heart health, and possibly brain longevity and health.

As a traditional part of the Mediterranean diet, it is intended to be enjoyed with a reasonable amount of food (e.g., a 5-ounce glass for women per day). Of course, it is not for everyone, and there are many other ways to eat and drink healthily for anyone who prefers to avoid wine for some reason.

11. Turmeric

Turmeric is the golden child of healthy food these days. It looks like ginger, but it's the color of sweet potatoes inside. Turmeric is a major ingredient in curry powders, and the active ingredient is curcumin, an anti-inflammatory and antioxidant compound. The body doesn't take it very well, so it's good that black pepper increases absorption by 2,000 percent.

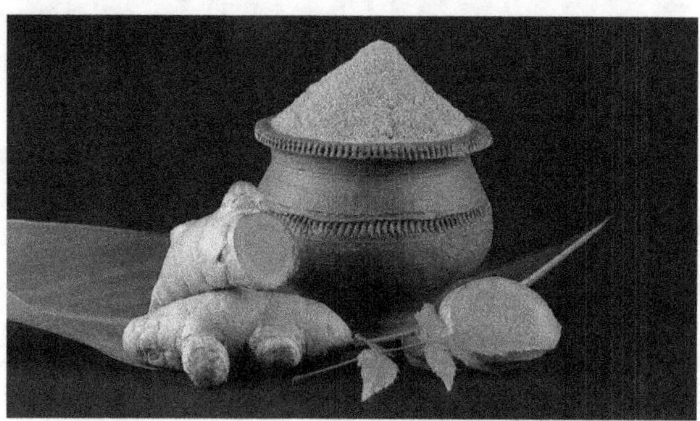

If you enjoy it with some healthy fat, the body can also absorb this fat-soluble antioxidant better. Make your own "golden milk" by whisking almond milk, coconut milk, turmeric, black pepper, ginger, and honey (optional) on low heat. Sprinkle cinnamon over it and enjoy it.

12. Medjool dates

The Sirtfood Diet won't tolerate sugar additives, but Medjool dates that have the gallic acid, polyphenols, and caffeic acid are acceptable. A study was done in 2011. You can read in the Journal of Nutrition discovered that eating dates did not significantly increase sugar levels of blood and was even connected with lesser rates of heart disease and diabetes.

If you throw back four dates, you have reached 30 percent of your daily fiber intake. They are also a good source of potassium, a nutritional deficiency in the American diet that helps with hydration, muscle contraction, and carbohydrate metabolism.

If you've kept your taste buds from overly sweet flavors, you may want to cut some dates into pieces and sparingly add them to savory dishes like curries, cereal salads, and pan sauces for fried chicken.

13. Capers

Capers are known to have potent anti-inflammatory benefits, giving lots of minerals, vitamins, and antioxidants. In terms of calories, they only yield 23-24 grams per serving of a hundred grams.

It can also provide high amounts of potassium, calcium, vitamin K, iron, copper, phytonutrients, and riboflavin. Rutin and Quercetin, the two main antioxidants found in capers also contains anti-carcinogenic, analgesic and antibacterial properties.

Rutin aids in the prevention and treatment of hemorrhoids, improvement om the circulation of the heart, and in the reduction of harmful cholesterol levels in the patient that are suffering obesity. Quercetin, on the other hand, prevents the growth of a tumor and helps in boosting the immune system. The ideal way to use capers is by using them to pasta, casseroles, and salads.

Chapter 8

The Sirt Food Juices and Smoothies

Both juices and whole foods are integral to the Sirtfood Diet. Here, we are talking about juices specifically made using a juicer and blenders and smoothie makers. For many, this will seem counterintuitive, on the basis that when something is juiced, the fiber is removed. But for leafy greens, this is exactly what we want.

The fiber from food contains what are called non-extractable polyphenols (or NEPPs). These are polyphenols, including sirtuin activators, that are attached to the fibrous part of the food and are only released when broken down by our friendly gut bacteria. By removing the fiber, we don't get the NEPPs and lose out on their goodness. But importantly, the NEPP content varies dramatically depending on the type of plant.

The NEPP content of foods like fruit, cereals, and nuts is significant, and these should be eaten whole (in strawberries, NEPPs provide more than 50 percent of the polyphenols!). But for leafy vegetables, the active ingredients in the Sirtfood juice, they are far lower despite a large bulk of fiber.

So, when it comes to leafy greens, we get maximum bang for our buck by juicing them and removing the low-nutrient fiber, meaning we can use much greater volumes and achieve a super-concentrated hit of sirtuin-activating polyphenols.

There is also another advantage of removing the fiber. Leafy greens contain a type of fiber called insoluble fiber, which has a scrubbing action in the digestive system. But when we eat too much of it, just like if we over scrub something, it can irritate and damage our gut lining.

That means green green-packed smoothies will be fiber overload for many people, potentially aggravating or even causing IBS (irritable bowel syndrome) and hindering our absorption of nutrients.

Having some of your Sirtfoods in juice form can also have big advantages when it comes to absorbing their goodness. For example, one of the ingredients we include in the green juice is matcha green tea.

When we consume the sirtuin activator EGCG, found in high levels in green tea, in drink form without food, its absorption is more than 65 percent higher.[10] We also find it interesting to note that when we ran blood tests on our own clients, switching from smoothies to green juices brought about dramatic increases in their levels of other essential nutrients such as magnesium and folic acid.

The crux of it all is that to really get those sirtuin genes firing for dramatic weight loss and health, and we need to build a diet that combines both juices and whole foods for maximum benefit.

As you familiarize yourself with the staples of the Sirtfood diet, you can also create your own juices and smoothies. Just avoid using any kind of processed sugar and be sure to load up in SIRT-activating greens and berries.

If you need to make a smoothie "smoother" add a teaspoon of olive oil, it will make it healthier and creamier! Smoothies are a great way to start the morning and ensure that you have your breakfast even if you are dashing out the door to get yourself to work and your children to school!

Even if they are best served immediately, you can prepare them the night before and leave them in the fridge for the morning, it will save you some extra time, and you won't be tempted to skip breakfast! *Here are the best green juices you can drink*

Lemony Green Juice

- 2 large green apples, cored and sliced
- 4 cups fresh kale leaves
- 4 tablespoons fresh parsley leaves
- 1 tablespoon fresh ginger, peeled
- 1 lemon, peeled
- ½ cup of filtered water
- Pinch of salt

Place all the ingredients in a blender and pulse until well combined.

Through a fine mesh strainer, strain the juice and transfer into 2 glasses.

Serve immediately.

Simple Celery Juice

- 8 celery stalks with leaves
- 2 tbsp fresh ginger, peeled
- 1 lemon, peeled
- ½ cup of filtered water
- Pinch of salt

Place all the ingredients in a blender and pulse until well combined.

Through a fine mesh strainer, strain the juice and transfer into 2 glasses.

Serve immediately.

Kale, apple, and celery juice

- 10 celery stalks with leaves
- 1 medium cucumber
- A handful of kale stems removes
- 1/2 apple with skin
- 1/2 organic lemon with peel
- 1-inch piece of ginger with peel

Wash all ingredients well and cut them to fit the feed chute of the juicer.

Then gradually pour into the feed chute and allow it to press out. If you prepare more juice in stock, the juice will last one or two days in the refrigerator.

Kale and orange juice	• 5 large oranges, peeled and sectioned • 2 bunches fresh kale	Add all ingredients into a juicer and extract the juice. Pour into 2 glasses and serve immediately.
Sweet green juice	• 10 celery stalks with leaves • 1 cup of pineapple, cut and peeled • 1/3 cup of parsley • 1/2 apple with skin • 1/2 organic lemon with peel	Wash all ingredients well and cut them to fit the feed chute of the juicer. Then gradually pour into the feed chute and allow it to press out. If you prepare more juice in stock, the juice will last one or two days in the refrigerator.
The greenest juice	• 1 kiwi, peeled, halved • ½ cup pre-pressed apple juice • ½ ripe pear, cored • 1 cup baby spinach leaves (pull off stems if you would like) • ¼ avocado pitted and scooped out	Simply juice all the ingredients until smooth. Serve immediately

Twice orange juice	• 2 oranges • 1 small grapefruit • 1 cup of freshly made carrots juice • 4 tbsp of buttermilk • 1 teaspoon of extra virgin olive oil	Press the grapefruit and oranges. Put all the ingredients and the pressed juices in a blender and mix until well blended. Serve immediately or slightly chilled.
Sweet red endive juice	• 1 whole red endive • 6 black figs, peeled • 4 tbsp of chokeberries (or blackcurrants) • 1 cup of yogurt • 1 tablespoon of honey or maple syrup	Put all the ingredients in a blender with 1 ½ cup of water and blend thoroughly. Serve immediately, or slightly chilled. Add extra honey to taste.
Kiwi cocktail	• 6 large Kiwis, peeled • 2 limes • All the seeds from 1 pomegranate • Ice cubes, to chill and serve	Press the limes and put the juice aside. Juice the pomegranate seeds. Blend the kiwis and the lime juice together, then add the pomegranate juice. Add ice to serve.

Watermelon Juice	• ½ cucumber halved • 2 cups baby kale (can remove stems if you like) • 2 cups of pre-cut watermelon chunks • 4 mint leaf	Add all to a blender and blend it very well. You cannot juice watermelon! Enjoy immediately
Cucumber and apple juice	• 3 large apples, cored and sliced • 2 large cucumbers, sliced • 4 celery stalks • 1 (1-inch) piece fresh ginger, peeled • 1 lemon, peeled	Add all ingredients into a juicer and extract the juice.
Matcha Green Tea Smoothie	• 2 bananas • 2 tsp Matcha green tea powder • 1/2 tsp vanilla bean (paste or scraped from a vanilla bean pod) • 1 ½ cups milk • 4-5 ice cubes • 2 tsp honey	Add all ingredients except the Matcha to a blender. Blend until smooth. (Make sure you have an ice-crusher blender, otherwise, leave out the ice and add later) When you are ready to serve to add the matcha and stir well. Let the Matcha dissolve for a few minutes before you serve

Green smoothie with berries	<ul><li>1 ripe banana</li><li>½ cup blackcurrants (take off stems)</li><li>10 baby kale leaves (take off stems)</li><li>2 tsp honey</li><li>1 cup freshly made green tea (dissolve honey first in tea then chill)</li><li>6 ice cubes</li></ul>	Dissolve the honey in the tea before you chill it. Cool first, and then blend all the ingredients in the blender until smooth. Serve chilled.
Green smoothie with grapefruit	<ul><li>1 grapefruit, peeled and deseeded</li><li>6 large kale leaves, destemmed</li><li>1 green or red apple, cored and destemmed.</li><li>1 carrot</li><li>½ cup of water (may use more or less for the texture that you like)</li></ul>	Place everything into a blender and blend until smooth. Add water if needed. Serve immediately or slightly chilled

Green smoothie with apples	• 1 green apple, cored and destemmed and sliced • 6 large kale leaves, destemmed • 1 orange, peeled • 1 stick of celery	Juice the orange separately in a blender and strain, unless you have a citrus juicer/press. Juice the celery, kale, and apple, mix together and stir, or add to a blender and pulse for a few seconds. Serve immediately or slightly chilled.
Creamy sunshine smoothie	• 1 avocado, pitted and scooped out • 1 banana • 5 leaves of kale, destemmed • ½ cup of pineapple juice • 8 oz. of coconut water	Place the liquids, then the fruits and veggies into a blender and blend until smooth. Serve immediately or slightly chilled.
Blueberries and coconut smoothie	• 1 banana, peeled and cut • 2 dry Medjool dates, without seeds • 1 tsp coconut oil • ½ cup of blueberries • 1 ½ cup of almond milk • ½ tsp of ground cinnamon • 2 tbsp of coconut flakes • 3 mint leaves	Put all the ingredients in a blender and blend thoroughly. Serve immediately or slightly chilled. For an extra kick, decorate with coconut flakes and mint leaves. For an extra kick, decorate with coconut flakes and mint leaves.

Creamy oats, greens, and blueberry smoothie	• 1 cup cold fat-free milk • 1 cup salad greens • ½ cup fresh frozen blueberries • ½ cup of frozen cooked oatmeal • 1 tbsp. sunflower seeds	In a powerful blender, blend all ingredients until smooth and creamy. Serve and enjoy.
Cranberry kale smoothie	• 75g (3 oz) strawberries • 50g (2 oz) kale • 120mls (4 fl oz) unsweetened cranberry juice • 1 teaspoon chia seeds • ½ teaspoon matcha powder	Place all of the ingredients into a blender and process until smooth. Add some crushed ice and a mint leaf or two for a really refreshing drink.
Mango and arugula smoothie	• 25g (1 oz) fresh rocket (arugula) • 150g (5 oz) fresh mango, peeled, de-stoned and chopped • 1 avocado, de-stoned and peeled • ½ teaspoon matcha powder • Juice of 1 lime	Place all of the ingredients into a blender with enough water to cover them and process until smooth. Add a few ice cubes and enjoy.

Banana and peanut butter green smoothie

- 1 cup chopped and packed Romaine lettuce
- 1 frozen medium banana
- 1 tbsp. all-natural peanut butter
- 1 cup cold almond milk

In a heavy-duty blender, add all ingredients.

Puree until smooth and creamy.

Serve and enjoy.

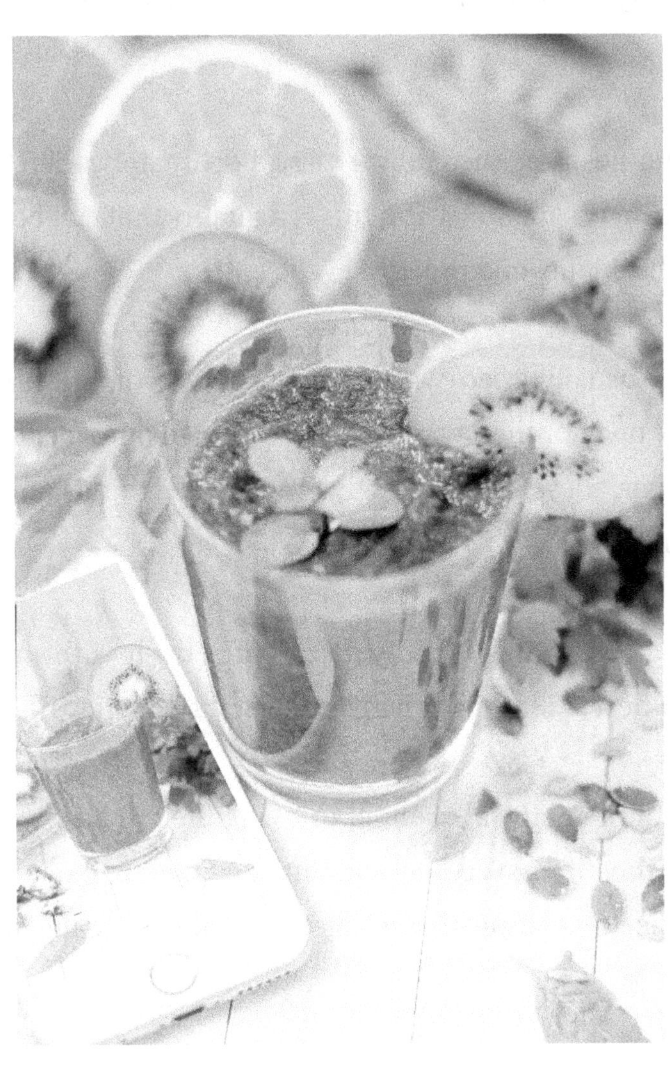

Chapter 9

How to Prepare your Mind to Diet
Be Mentally Tough

Are you able to prepare yourself up and adjust to circumstances when life knocks you down? Or are you totally overwhelmed by minimal confidence in your capability to tackle the challenges?

If you're in the latter position, then don't worry. Fortunately, there are numerous practical strategies to build resilience, mental-wise; this is a quality that can be acquired and improved through hard work, discipline, and practice.

One's resilience is usually tried when circumstances of life are changing out of our expectations and may turn for the worse — such as a loved one's death, losing a job or ending a relationship. However, these challenges give the chance to rise and have the strength and be stronger than ever.

Mental strength is an individual's ability to cope effectively with stresses and obstacles and to make most of their best skills, regardless of the situations they find themselves in.

Developing strength mentally is essential to living life the best way you can. Even as we make our way into the fitness center and lift weights to make our muscles stronger, physically, we also need to improve our mental state by using mental techniques and resources.

Good mental wellbeing leads towards a life we love and allow us to have successful social interactions and good self-esteem. This also helps to try new things, manage risks, and coping with any hard situation that we might experience in life. We have to construct our strength mentally to be mentally fit! This is a thing that develops over time when individuals make development a main priority. If we want to experience gains in mental health, we need to upgrade good mental habits like to practice gratitude.

In the same sense, to see good physical effects, we must learn to steer away from unhealthy habits, such as consuming junk food. We can all become mentally stronger; the secret is to keep your mental muscles practiced and exercised — just like you are training your muscles to be physically good.

Mental Toughness pertains to the power to be storing despite the presence of adversity, to remain focused and determined, despite the hardships and challenges you might face. A mentally tough individual sees challenges and distress as a chance rather than a danger and has confidence.

You must have some degree of resilience to be mentally tough, but not all resilient people are mentally tough. If you realize it as a metaphor, the mountain would be resilient, while mental toughness could be one of the strategies for climbing that mountain.

Resilience helps you survive, and mental toughness helps you to thrive. Mental resilience begins when you want to consider what's going through your mind without directly connecting with certain thoughts or feelings. Then, find the resolution to evoke positive thoughts about the present situation.

That is the extent of your personal attention and trust. Being high on the scale of the commitments means that being able to set targets successfully and to reach them regularly without getting disturbed.

A high level of commitment indicates that you are good at establishing successful routines and habits. Below the Commitment, scale indicates that you may find it hard to set goals and prioritize them, or to adapt routines or habits that indicate success. Certain people or conflicting interests could easily confuse you too.

The scales of Control and Dedication together reflect the Endurance aspect of Mental Toughness. It also takes concentration and the capability to set patterns and goals to put you back on the path that you have chosen. Being high on the scale of the challenge means you are motivated to reach your best version, and you see obstacles, change, and difficulty as means to improve rather than bad events; you have more chances to be resilient and agile.

Being low on the scale of the challenge means you might perceive change as something challenging and step back from new or challenging situations because you are scared to fail.

It's your belief in yourself and that mindset in influencing other people. To be able to step up on the scale of confidence is to assume that you can complete tasks effectively and take setbacks step by step while preserving habit and even improving your resolve. Being low on the scale of confidence means you are easily disappointed with failure and don't believe that you can or have an influence on others.

The scales of Challenge and Trust together embody the Confidence, part of the definition of Mental Toughness. It is sensible because you are more likely to turn challenges into positive results if you are sure in your own self and your skills and communicate easily with others.

As with building mental power, it takes self-awareness and determination to grow mental toughness. In general, mentally strong people tend to gain more than mentally weak people and experience a greater degree of contentment.

Be Consistent

It is important to be consistent if you want to bring about some positive change in your life. If you are looking to kick some serious ass and become world-class, it's also a must-have skill. When you want to change something in your life (and I bet you are!), here are keys that will motivate you to be more reliable. You become fixed on a specific goal, like composing a novel or just lose weight. You ride that wave of motivation for the first few days. You are showing up, doing the work, moving forward.

But the novelty then wears off. You start doing the practice of skipping. You cease to be consistent. A day here and a day there, and you haven't written a word for days.

To maximize your chances of success, tied to changes in personality. You don't want to attain it; you want to become. You are the one who's writing—a good person who does clean eating and exercise. You handle personal finances well.

Read Inspiration Studies

In a culture obsessed with assessing talent and ability, the essential role of inspiration is often overlooked. By encouraging us to overcome our ordinary experiences and limitations, Imagination awakens us to new possibilities.

Inspiration propels a person to possibility from apathy and transforms the way we view our own capabilities. Inspiration can occasionally be overlooked due to its elusive nature. Its history of being treated as divine or supernatural has not helped the situation. But creativity can be triggered, recorded, and exploited, and it has a significant impact on important outcomes in life.

Compared to typical daily life experiences, motivation includes elevated levels of positive influence and participation in projects and lower levels of negative effect. However, inspiration isn't the same as a positive effect. Compared to being in an excited and enthusiastic state, people entering an inspired state (thinking about an earlier moment they were motivated) register higher levels about spirituality and meaning, and lower levels of positive power, controllability, and self-responsibility.

Although the positive impact is triggered when anyone progresses toward their immediate, conscious goals and motivation that is more closely linked to awakening to something new, greater, or more important: the transcendence of past concerns.

Inspiration was more closely linked to the future than to happiness with the present. The degree to which inspiration persisted has been explained by self-reported intention rates and lifetime gratitude.

Such results suggest that inspiration has essential importance, which, given the natural and evocative characteristics of inspiration, may lead someone to have pressure felt by them to get inspired and unable to do so. But you shouldn't push yourself to get motivated. Such primary research results indicate that there is no need for inspiration – it happens. Knowing this will set you free from the need to inspire.

This does not mean that inspiration is entirely beyond your control. Opposite to the entire divine or mythical source of inspiration, I believe inspiration is a great thought of an unexpected conversation between the information you receive from the world and your current knowledge, and There are more things you can do to make inspiration more likely to happen. Research demonstrates very clearly that planning is a crucial element ("work mastery").

Although inspiration is not the same as effort, the effort is a necessary condition for inspiration, which prepares the mind for an inspiring experience. Openness to Experience and positive impact is also significant because having an open mind and an approach-oriented mindset can make you more likely to be conscious of the inspiration when it arrives. Small milestones are also critical because they can raise motivation by setting a successful and imaginative process in motion.

Chapter 10

Phase 1: 7 Pounds in Seven Days

Welcome to Phase 1 of the Sirtfood Diet. This is the hyper success stage, where you'll make a tremendous step towards showing up at a slimmer and increasingly thin body. Follow our first a tiny bit at a time rule and use the good plans obliged you.

Despite our famous seven-day policy, we even have a sans meat version, which is reasonable for the two veggie sweethearts and vegans. Don't hesitate to go with whichever one you like.

What's To Expect

This last for 7 days, plus it is divided up. Throughout the first 3 days, you should possess three Sirtfood green juices and also something routine meal which is full of Sirtfoods--for an overall total of 1000 calories each day. On days four through seven, you should have two juices and 2 daily meals for a total of 1,500 calories each day.

During Phase 1, you may get the full benefits of our clinically shown methodology for dropping 7 kilos in seven days. In any case, audit this contains muscle gain, so don't get hung up just with the numbers at the scales, nor should you begin checking yourself reliably. When in doubt, we much of the time watch the levels creeping up inside the past couple of extensive stretches of Phase 1 considering muscle gain, all the while as waistlines hold to wither.

That is the explanation we need you to mull over the scales, yet at this point, not be overseen through them. Take a gander at the way wherein you search inside the mirror, how your articles of clothing are getting, or whether you have to move an intent on your belt. These are through and through large signs of the more considerable changes in your edge structure.

Think about different changes, too, for instance, in your vibe of flourishing, your quality levels, and how clean your pores and skin look. You may even get estimations of your standard cardiovascular and metabolic prosperity performed at your local medication store to see changes in things like your circulatory strain, glucose levels, and blood fat exhaustive of cholesterol and triglycerides.

Remember, weight decrease aside, the creation of Sirtfoods into your eating routine is a serious step forward in making your cells better and increasingly noticeable impenetrable to infection, putting you up for a lifetime of uncommon wellbeing.

Directions for Phase

To make Phase 1 as direct cruising as could be reasonable in light of the current situation, we'll manual you through the complete seven-day plan every day thus, together with the lowdown at the Sirtfood green press and smooth-to follow, superb ideas consistently.

Stage 1 of the Sirtfood Diet relies upon amazing scenes:

Days 1 to a couple are the most focused, and all through this period, you can eat up to the furthest reaches of 1,000 calories consistently, including:
- 3 x Sirtfood fresh squeezes
- 1 x basic supper

Days four to 7 will see your meals utilization impact to a restrict of 1,500 calories reliably, including:
- 2 x Sirtfood green juices
- 2 x guideline food

There are only several game plans for following the food schedule. In the long run, it's generally getting it into your lifestyle and round ordinary living for postponed fulfillment.

Regardless, straightforwardly here are a few essential yet significant impact suggestions for accomplishing the enchanting outcome:

1. Get a Good Juicer: Juicing is an imperative bit of the Sirtfood Diet, and a juicer is one among the best endeavors you'll make for your health (to recap why to see page 68). While records ought to be the understanding variable, two or three juicers are additional earth-shattering at expelling the juice from green verdant veggies and herbs, with the Breville brand being among the best of the routinely available juicers we have endeavored.

2. Game plan Is Key: From the abundance of analysis, we have made them thing, is clear: individuals who orchestrated early have been the best. Become more acquainted with the parts and plans and stock up on what you need. With everything on the side
Formed and arranged, you'll be stunned at how clean the whole method is.

3. Save Time: If you're tight for time, set up wisely. Meals may be made the night sooner than. Juices may be made in mass and kept inside the cooler for up to two or three days (or longer in the cooler) before their degrees of sirtuin-starting enhancements start to drop. Shield it from light, and handiest incorporate the matcha while you are equipped to eat it.

4. Eat Early: It is higher to eat earlier inside the day, and food and juices need to ideally now not be eaten up later than 7 p.m. (to recap why to see page 71); yet as time goes on the eating routine is proposed to t with your lifestyle, and past-due eaters despite everything get stunning benet.

5. Space Out the Juices: To light up the ingestion of the green juices, they ought to be eaten up as a base an hour sooner than or two hours after dinner and spread out in the long run of the day, rather than having them unnecessarily near together.
6. Eat till satisfied Sirtfoods can have electrifying results on hunger (see pages 31–33), and two or three people might be full before finishing them

food. Check out your body and eat until you're satisfied as opposed to convincing all the suppers down. As the deep Okinawans state, "Hara Hachi bu," which, for the most part, deciphers as "Eat until you are 80 rates full."

7. Welcome the Journey: Don't raise got to an acceptable level close to the end reason; rather, live mindful of the outing. This weight decrease plan is connected to lauding dinners in the sum of its wonder, for its prosperity benefits at any rate likewise for the satisfaction and joy it brings. Research suggests that after we hold our minds centered at the course in the tendency to the final objective, we will undoubtedly succeed.

What to Drink

As agreeably because of the proposed step by step servings of natural juices, you can eat up various juices straightforwardly at the end of Phase 1. These ought to be noncaloric liquids, in a perfect world essential water, dark espresso, and fresh tea. In case your normal tendency is for dim or basic beverages, sense segregated to join those also. Soft drink pops and regular item squeezes

Are abandoned. Or maybe, in case you need to jazz things up, try including two or three slice strawberries to regardless or shimmering water to make your Sirtfood-saturated wellbeing drink. Spare it inside the cooler for a few hours, and you'll have a pleasantly restoring choice as opposed to soft drink pops and crushes.

One factor to be aware of is that we do now not propose unforeseen titanic changes as per your customary espresso usage. Caffeine withdrawal signs can make you experience loathsome for more than one day; comparatively, enormous augmentations can be immense for those interestingly sensitive with the effects of caffeine.

We, in like manner, advocate that coffee is inebriated dull, without including milk, because of the truth a couple of researchers have found that the choice of milk can diminish the maintenance of the beneficial sirtuin-ordering vitamins. The undefined has been found for natural tea, disregarding the way that including a few lemon crush indeed will extend the ingestion of its sirtuin-impelling nutrients.

Do consider that that is the hyper-achievement stage, and remember that you should be helped by strategy for the way that it's far for multi-week best, you ought to be reasonably extra prepared. During the present week, we contain alcohol, inside the kind of red wine, in any case, similar to a cooking fixing.

The Sirt Food Green Juice

The natural juice is an essential bit of Phase 1 of the Sirtfood Diet. All the substances are unbelievable Sirtfoods, and in each sauce, you get a staggering combined beverage of unique blends in with apigenin, kaempferol, luteolin, quercetin, and EGCG that coordinate to replace to your sirtuin characteristics and advance fat hardship.

To that, we've introduced lemon, as its home-developed sharpness has been shown to shield, balance out, and improve the maintenance of the drink's sirtuin-inciting supplements. We've moreover incorporated a scramble of apple and ginger for the season.

Both of these are in this manner optional. Various people and that once they may be acquainted with the sort of the juice, they neglect the apple all things considered.

Sirt Green Juice Recipe (Serving 1)

- ✓ Two significant bundles (around 75g or 21/2 oz.) kale a gigantic bundle
- ✓ (30 g or 1 ounce) arugula a tiny pack
- ✓ (around 5g or ¼ ounce) at-leaf parsley
- ✓ 2 to 3 tremendous celery stems (51/2 oz or 150g, for instance, leaves 1/2 medium green apple half of-to 1-inch (1 to 2.5 cm)
- ✓ bit of sparkling ginger juice of half of lemon

✓ 1/2-degree teaspoon matcha powder*

*Days 1 to 3 of Phase 1: passed on best to the rest juices of the day;

Days 4 to 7 of Phase 1: passed on to the two juices

Note that all the while, as in our pilot organic, the whole of what fragments have been weighed out correctly as recorded, our acknowledge is that bundle gauges work inconceivably agreeably. They better tailor the enhancement that adds up to an individual's body size. Higher individuals ordinarily will, by and large, have more fabulous hands, and along these lines get a moderately higher measure of Sirtfood supplements to organize their body size and the opposite way around for more diminutive people.

• Combine the greens (Arugula, kale, parsley) by then squeeze them. We and that juicers can truly differentiate in their effectiveness at crushing verdant vegetables, and maybe there's a need to rejoice the leftovers sooner than proceeding onward to the different parts. The desire is to grow moreover with around two oz. or then again near 1/4 cup (50ml) of juice from the greens.

• Now crush the celery, apple, and ginger.

• You can strip the lemon and arranged it through the juicer; likewise, in any case, we and it much less hard to undeniably press the lemon by methods for hand into the juice. By this stage, you must have cycle 1 cup (250ml) of fluid inside and out, possibly insignificantly extra.

• It is ideal while the sauce is made and arranged to serve which you incorporate the matcha. Pour a modest amount of the liquid.

Chapter 11

Phase 2 of the Sirtfood Diet

Congratulations on completing Sirtfood Diet Step 1! You should already have excellent results of fat loss and not only appear slimmer and more toned but also feel revitalized and re-energized. Okay, now what?

Having seen these sometimes-incredible changes ourselves, we realize how much you're going to want to see much better results, not just retain all those advantages. Sirtfoods are, after all, designed to eat for life. The problem is how you adapt what you learned in Phase 1 into your regular dietary practice.

That is precisely what inspired us to develop a fourteen-day maintenance plan designed to help you make the transition from Phase 1 to your more usual dietary regimen, thus helping to

What to Expect

You should maintain the weight loss results through Phase 2 and continue to lose weight gradually. Also, the one striking thing we've seen with the Sirtfood Diet is that most or all of the weight people lose is from fat and that many put some muscle on. So, we would like to warn you again not to measure your success solely based on the numbers. Look in the mirror to see if you look leaner and more toned, see how well your clothes fit and lap up the compliments you'll get from others.

Note that just as weight loss occurs, the health benefits will increase. In implementing the fourteen-day maintenance plan, you are helping to lay the foundations for a lifelong health future.

Step by step Process of Phase 2

The key to success in this process is having your diet packed full of Sirtfoods. We've put together a seven-day meal schedule for you to adapt to make it as easy as possible, with tasty family-friendly meals, filled with Sirtfoods every day to the rafters. Now what you need to do is to implement the Seven Day Program twice to fulfill Phase 2's fourteen days.

On each of fourteen days, your diet will consist of:

- Three times balanced sirtfood meals

- 1-time sirtfood green juice

- 1 – 2 times optional sirtfood snacks

Also, when you have to eat those, there are no strict laws. Be agile throughout every day and suit them. Two basic thumb-rules are:

- Take sirtfood green juice either in the morning or at least half an hour before breakfast.

- Try your best to make dinner by 7 PM.

How to Portion

In Phase 2, our attention is not on calorie counting. For the average person, this is not a practical approach or even a good one over the long term.

Instead, we concentrate on healthy servings, really well-balanced meals, and most notably, filling up on Sirtfoods so that you can continue to benefit from their fat-burning and health-promoting impact.

We've even designed the meals in the plan to make them satiate, making you stay full for longer. This, coupled with Sirtfoods' innate appetite-regulating power, ensures you're not going to spend the next 14 days feeling thirsty, but rather comfortably fulfilled, well-fed, and highly well-nourished.

Just like in Phase 1, try to listen and be driven by your appetite. When you prepare meals according to our guidelines and notice that you are easily full before you finish a meal, then stop eating is perfectly fine!

What You Can Drink

During Phase 2, you'll need to include one green juice every day. This is to keep you top with high Sirtfoods prices.

Just like in Phase 1, you will easily absorb other fluids in Phase 2. Our preferred beverages contain remaining plain water, bottled flavored water, coffee, and green tea. Whether black or white tea is your preference, feel free to enjoy it.

The same goes for herbal teas. The best news is that during Phase 2, you will enjoy the occasional bottle of red wine. Due to its content of sirtuin-activating polyphenols, particularly resveratrol and piceatannol, red wine is a sirtfood that makes it the best choice of alcoholic beverage.

However, with alcohol itself causing adverse effects on our fat cells, restraint is still safest, so we suggest restricting the drink to one glass of red wine with a meal for two to three days a week in Phase 2.

Returning to Three Meals

You enjoyed only one or two meals per day during Phase 1 and allowed you plenty of versatility when you eat your meals. As we are now back to a more normal routine and the well-tested practice of three meals a day, learning about breakfast is a good time.

We are eating a good breakfast sets, us on for the day, raising our levels of energy and focus. Eating early holds our blood sugar and fat rates in balance, in terms of our metabolism. The breakfast is a good thing that is pointed out by some studies, usually showing that people who eat breakfast often are less prone to overweight.

The explanation for this is because of our internal clocks inside. Our bodies are asking us to feed early in expectation of when we will be most busy and need food. Yet, as many as a third of us will miss breakfasts on any given day. It's a classic symptom in our crazy modern life, and the feeling is there's simply not enough time to eat properly. But as you will see, with the nifty breakfasts we have laid out for you here, nothing could be further from the truth.

Whether it's the Sirtfood smoothie that can be drunk on the go, the premade Sirt muesli, or the quick and easy Sirtfood scrambled eggs/tofu, finding those extra few minutes in the morning will reap dividends not only for your day but for your longer-term weight and health.

With Sirtfoods functioning to overcharge our energy levels, there's, even more, to learn from getting a hit from them early in the morning to continue your day. This is done not only by consuming a Sirtfood-rich meal but above all by including the green juice, which we suggest you have either first thing in the morning — at least thirty minutes before breakfast— or mid-morning.

We get a lot of reports from our personal experience of people who first consume their green juice and don't feel hungry for a few hours afterward. If this is the impact it's having on you, taking a couple of hours until having breakfast is perfectly fine. Just don't miss this one.

Instead, with a good breakfast, you should kick off your day, then wait two to three hours to have the green juice. Be versatile, and just go with anything that suits you.

Snacking

You should keep it when it comes to snacking or quit it. There is a long debate on whether consuming regular, smaller meals is better for weight loss, or just keeping to three balanced meals a day. The fact is, that does not matter.

The way we've designed the maintenance menu for you means you're going to eat three well-balanced Sirtfood-rich meals a day, and you may notice that you don't need a snack. But maybe you've been busy with the kids in the classroom, working out or dashing about and need something to take you into the next meal.

And if that "little something" is going to give you a whammy of Sirtfood nutrients and taste delicious, then it's happy days. This is why we created our "Sirtfood bites." These smart little snacks are a genuinely guilt-free treat made entirely from Sirtfoods: dates, walnuts, cocoa, extra virgin olive oil, and turmeric. We recommend eating one, or a maximum of two, per day for the days when you require them.

Sirtifying Your Meal

We saw that the only consistent diets are those of participation, not exclusion. Yet real success goes beyond this— the diet has to be consistent with living in modern days. Whether it's the ease of meeting the demands of our hectic lives or fitting in with our position at dinner parties as to the bon vivant, the way we eat should be trouble-free. You will appreciate your svelte body and beautiful smile, rather than thinking about the demands and limitations of kooky products.

What makes Sirtfoods so great is that they are available, common, and simple to include in your diet. Below, when you bridge the gap between step 1 and daily feeding, you can lay the foundations for a modern, better lifelong eating strategy.

The key principle is what we term the meals "Sirtifying." This is where we take popular meals, including many traditional classics, and we retain all the great taste with some smart modifications and easy Sirtfood inclusions but attach a lot of goodness to that. You'll see just how quickly this is done in Phase 2.

Highlights include our tasty smoothie Sirtfood for the ultimate on-the-go breakfast in a time-consuming environment and the easy turn from wheat to buckwheat to add extra flavor and zip to the much-loved pasta comfort food. While a classic, famous dishes such as chili con Carne and curry don't even need much improvement, with Sirtfood bonanzas providing traditional recipes.

Yet who has said that fast food means bad health? If you prepare something yourself, we mix the true vivid tastes of a pizza and through the shame. There's no need to say goodbye to indulgence yet, as our smothered pancakes with berries and dark chocolate sauce have demonstrated.

It's not even a treat, it's breakfast, and for you it's perfect. Simple changes: you keep eating the things that you enjoy when maintaining healthy weight and well-being. And that is Sirtfoods, the culinary movement.

After the Diet

You may replicate these two phases as much you desired for additional weight loss.

However, you are advised to continue "sirtifying" your diet at the end of completing these phases by including sirtfoods frequently into your meals.

There are variations of Sirtfood Diet manuals that has several recipes rich in sirtfoods. You can also add sirtfoods in your foods as a snack or in recipes you have previously use. In addition, you are advised to continue taking the green juice daily.

In this manner, the Sirtfood Diet will be more of a way of lifestyle adjustment than a one-time diet.

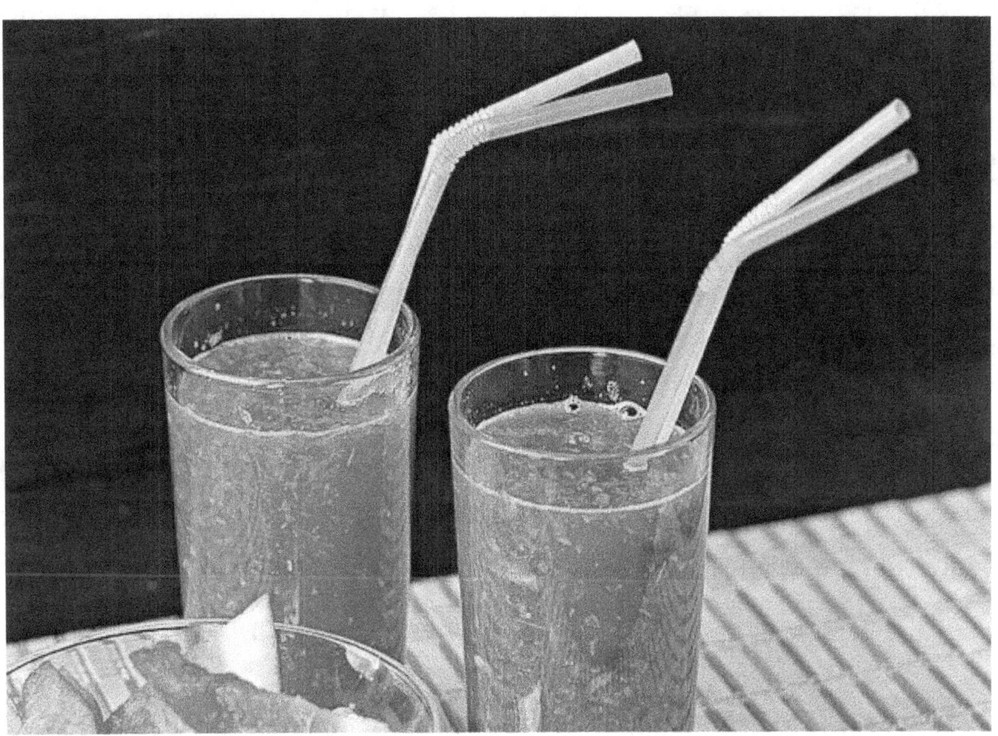

Chapter 12

7 -Day Meal Plan

The diet is subdivided into two phases. Phase 1 is called the 'hyper success phase' of 7 days, incorporating a Sirtfood-rich diet with mild calorie restriction, and Phase 2 is the 'maintenance phase' of 14 days, where you maintain your weight loss without reducing calories. Intake of calories is limited to calories of 1000 over the first three days (so, even more than on a five ratio two during the day you will do fasting). The diet will consist of 3 green juices rich in sirtfood and one meal rich in sirtfood and two cubes of dark chocolate.

Calories are increased to calories of 1500 over the remaining four days, and the diet includes two sirtfood-rich meals and two sirtfood-rich green juices daily. You are not permitted to drink any alcohol during Phase 1, but you are free to drink soda, tea, coffee, and green tea. Phase 2 is not about limiting calories.

Each day includes three sirtfood-rich meals and one green juice, plus one or two Sirtfood bite snacks, if necessary. You can drink red wine in Phase 2 but in moderation (recommendation is 2-3 glasses of red wine per week), as well as beer, tea, coffee, and green tea.

The Sirtfood Diet is not intended as a onetime diet you'll do but more towards a change of lifestyle. You are advised to continue consuming a meal plan full of Sirtfoods after you've completed the first three weeks and continue to drink your everyday green juice.

We recommend that phases 1 and 2 can be done again if and when required for a health boost, or if things have gone off the way. You can do this plan for up to two weeks, after which it's all about changing your lifestyle accordingly. There are no restrictions – aim to include as many sirt foods as you can in your diet, which will help your skin feel safer, healthier, and smarter.

The Sirtfood Diet is not intended as a one-off 'diet' but rather as a way of life. You are advised to continue consuming a diet rich in Sirtfoods after you've completed the first three weeks and continue to drink your daily green juice.

The phases 1 and 2 can be repeated if required for a health boost if things have gone a little off track. However, after completing these phases, you are prompted to carry on "sirtifying" your diet by regularly incorporating sirtfoods into the meals you are preparing. You may also add the Sirt food in your meal plan as a snack or in the recipes you've already used.

We have given a better compilation of Sirtfood recipes, which can be followed. Furthermore, you are highly recommended to keep on consuming green juice every day. Thus, the Sirtfood Diet will become more of a change in lifestyle than a diet done only once.

After -Diet Meal Plan Guide

Here's our recommended meal structure, which will help you maintain the effects of your Sirt Diet. You may choose among the recipes in our cookbook, which has many options, making you have a variety in flavors and type of food you eat.

Each day you will consume

- Three times balanced sirtfood meals

- 1-time sirtfood green juice

- 1 – 2 times optional sirtfood snacks

Should You Go for Sirtfood or Not?

The Sirtfood Diet supports fruit and vegetable consumption that detoxes your body to prevent harm. Many people are also attracted to the fact that you can eat chocolate and drink red wine in your diet! Hence it is advisable to turn to sirtfood diet, which is a new regime in diet foods. The 23 top Sirtfoods form the foundation of the Mediterranean diet and the Japanese diet, where obesity and disease inhabitants are lower. Five times as many foods are eaten in the Japanese as in the Western world.

It's important to identify healthy eating and exercise regimes that are practicable, do not take away from anything that you like and don't require you to practice throughout the week with an estimated 650 million obese adults worldwide. That's precisely what the Sirtfood diet does.

The idea is that certain foods activate the "skinny gene" paths, often triggered by fasting and workouts.

The best thing is that some foods and beverages, including dark chocolate and red wine, contain the chemicals known as polyphenols, which activate the genes that imitate exercise and quickness.

Diet to Activate Sirtuins and Promote Health

It's no coincidence that people with a long span of life and the healthiest group of people around the world eat diets that are rich in sirtuin-activating foods, like in Asia or Mediterranean countries. Their diet includes vegetables and fruits, even wine and olive oil rich in polyphenol. For Asian people, ingredients such as soya beans and green tea are rich in isoflavones and epigallactins.

Getting this health developing food into your meal plan is actually pretty easy. It can be included in many diets and even utilized them to make Sirt-rich meals.

Here are some great ideas you can start with:

- Instead of other oils, use olive oil for roasting veggies or frying. Make use of it to make salad dressing as well

- Make Sure to have a jar of olives in your pantry to snack on and put them to cooked meals and salads. You can also make a tapenade as topping for your toast.

- Try to drink green tea as a substitute for coffee and usual tea. Add a squeeze of lemon for extra taste

- Miso alternatively can be utilized rather than readymade stock or cubes to flavor soups and stews. Milder light-colored miso may also serve as a spread. Miso soup also can be a great snack or soft meal if presented with salad or bread.

- Include tempeh or tofu to stir-fries. Mix soft tofu into soups, immerse, and desserts with cream.

- Put black currant and blueberries to your juice, muesli, and smoothies and. Fresh yogurt, as well as fresh berries, ensure a healthy dessert or snack

- Take your greens, broccoli, and outstanding cabbage support to meals and can also be included in stews, curries, stir-fries, and casseroles.

- Enrich up your life with spices like turmeric. Don't restrict your input of seasonings to curries, include them to vegetables and grains.

- Include cacao powder to desserts and smoothies too. Dredge cacao nibs on salads or include to trail mixes.

- Apples are the ideal handy snack. Make sure you have one with you most times.

- Buckwheat macaroni can be made as a delicious gluten complimentary option to buckwheat flour, and wheat pasta can also be made in baked products or to stiffer sauces. Buckwheat is also a great alternative that goes well with salads combined with toasted nuts and roasted vegetables.

Chapter 13

Sirtfood Recipes

KALE TURMERIC SCRAMBLE

Ingredients:

- 2 eggs
- 1/8 teaspoon ground turmeric
- Salt and black pepper
- ½ fl oz water
- 1 fl oz olive oil
- ½ cup fresh kale, chopped

Directions:

1. In a bowl, add the eggs, turmeric, salt, black pepper, and water and with a whisk, beat until foamy. In a wok, heat the oil over medium heat.
2. Add the egg mixture and mix. Immediately, lower down the heat to medium-low and cook for about 1–2 minutes, stirring frequently.
3. Mix in the kale and cook for about 3–4 minutes, stirring frequently.
4. Put away from the heat and serve immediately.

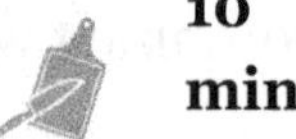 **10 mins** 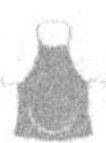 **5 mins**  1

Calories: 153 - Fat: 9.4g
Carbs: 25.1g - Protein: 9.6g

Ingredients:

- 1 cup buckwheat, rinsed
- 8 fl oz unsweetened almond milk
- 8 fl oz water
- ½ teaspoon ground cinnamon
- ½ teaspoon vanilla extract
- 1–2 tablespoons raw honey
- ¼ cup fresh blueberries

Directions:

1. In a pan, add all the ingredients (except honey and blueberries) over medium-high heat and bring to a boil.
2. Now, reduce the heat to low and simmer, covered for about 10 minutes. Stir in the honey and remove from the heat.
3. Set aside, covered, for about 5 minutes.
4. With a fork, fluff the mixture, and transfer into serving bowls.
5. Top with blueberries and serve.

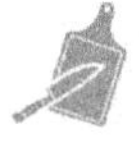 **10 mins** 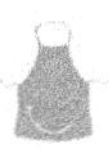 **15 mins** 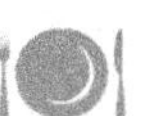 1

Calories: 297 - Fat: 3.8g
Carbs: 28.5g - Protein: 10.4g

Ingredients:

- ½ fl oz Coconut oil
- ½ piece Red onion
- 2 cloves Garlic
- 5 ½ oz (150 g) Broccoli
- ½ piece Zucchini
- 15 fl oz (450 ml) vegetable broth

Directions:

1. Finely chop the onion and garlic, cut the broccoli into florets, and the zucchini into slices.
2. Melt the coconut oil in a soup pot and fry the onion with the garlic.
3. Cook the zucchini for a few minutes.
4. Add broccoli and vegetable broth and simmer for about 5 minutes.
5. Puree the soup with a hand blender and season with salt and pepper.

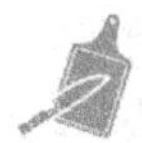 5 mins 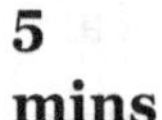 10 mins 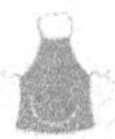 1 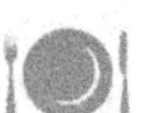  Calories: 178 - Fat: 14.4g – Fiber: 5.7g
Carbs: 10.57g - Protein: 2.1g

SALMON AND SPINACH QUICHE

Ingredients:

- 21 oz (600 g) frozen leaf spinach
- 1 clove of garlic
- 1 onion
- 5 ½ oz (150 g) frozen salmon fillets
- 7 oz (200 g) smoked salmon
- 1 small bunch of dill
- 1 untreated lemon
- 1 ⅓ oz (50 g) butter
- 7 oz (200 g) sour cream
- 3 eggs
- Salt, pepper, nutmeg
- 1 pack of puff pastry

Directions:

1. Let the spinach thaw and squeeze well. Peel the garlic and onion and cut into fine cubes. Cut the salmon fillet into cubes 0,4 – 0,6 in (1-1.5 cm) thick. Cut the smoked salmon into strips. Wash the dill, pat dry and chop.

2. Wash the lemon with hot water, dry, rub the zest finely with a kitchen grater and squeeze the lemon. Heat the butter in a pan. Sweat the garlic and onion cubes in it for approx. 2-3 minutes.

3. Add spinach and sweat briefly. Add sour cream, lemon juice and zest, eggs and dill and mix well. Season with salt, pepper, and nutmeg.

4. Preheat the oven to 390° F (200° C) top/bottom heat (350° F (180° C) convection). Grease a springform pan and roll out the puff pastry in it and pull up on edge. Prick the dough with a fork (so that it doesn't rise too much).

5. Pour in the spinach and egg mixture and smooth out. Spread salmon cubes and smoked salmon strips on top. The quiche in the oven (grid, middle inset) about 30-40 min. Yellow gold bake.

 **15 mins** 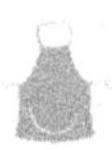 **30/40 mins** 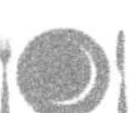 2

Calories: 315 - Fat: 4.7g
Carbs: 45g - Protein: 8.4g

Ingredients:

- 3½ oz (100 g) red chicory or yellow if not available
- 5 oz (140 g) tinned tuna flakes in brine, drained
- 3 ½ oz (100 g) cucumber
- 1 oz (30 g) rocket arugula
- 6 pitted black olives
- 2 hard-boiled eggs, peeled and quartered
- 2 tomatoes, chopped
- 2 tablespoons fresh parsley, chopped
- 1 red onion, chopped
- 1 stalk of celery
- 1 tablespoon capers
- 1 fl oz (30 ml) vinaigrette

Directions:

1. Place the tuna, cucumber, olives, tomatoes, onion, chicory, celery, parsley and rocket arugula into a bowl.
2. Pour in the vinaigrette and toss the salad in the dressing.
3. Serve onto plates and scatter the eggs and capers on top.

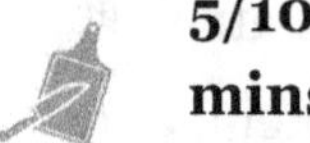 **5/10 mins** 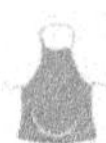 **0 mins**  1 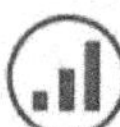 Calories: 309 - Fat: 12.2g – Fiber: 6g
Carbs: 25.76g - Protein: 26.72g

Ingredients:

- ¹/3 oz (20 g) Ghee
- 1 fl oz (30 ml) Olive oil
- 2 pieces Leek
- 5 fl oz (150 ml) vegetable broth

- fresh parsley
- 1 tablespoon fresh oregano
- 1 tablespoon Pine nuts (roasted)

Directions:

1. Chop the leeks and herbs finely. In a pan, roast the pine nuts over medium heat.
2. Then in another pan, melt the olive oil and ghee together. Put in the leeks and let it cook until golden brown for 5 minutes, stirring constantly.
3. Add the vegetable broth and cook for another 10 minutes until the leek is tender.
4. Stir in the herbs and sprinkle the pine nuts on the dish just before serving.

 5 mins  10/15 mins  1

Calories: 95 - Fat: 4.84g – Fiber: 4.1g
Carbs: 12.61g - Protein: 1.35g

Ingredients:

- 7 oz (200 g) new potatoes, split
- 2 garlic cloves, squashed
- 1 teaspoon turmeric powder
- ¼ teaspoon dried coriander
- ¼ teaspoon stew drops or powder
- ¼ teaspoon ginger powder
- 3 oz (80 g) container of coconut milk
- 1 tbsp tomato paste
- 4½ oz (120 g) container of slashed tomatoes
- Salt and pepper
- 4 ½ oz (120 g) quinoa
- 3½ oz (100 g) container of chickpeas, depleted and flushed
- 2⅔ oz (75 g) spinach

Directions:

1. Spot the potatoes in a dish of cold water and bring to the boil; at that point, let them cook for around 25 minutes until you can undoubtedly stick a blade through them. Channel them well.

2. Spot the potatoes in an enormous skillet and include the turmeric, garlic, bean stew, coriander, coconut milk, ginger, tomato paste, and tomatoes. Let it boil, then season with pepper and salt at that point include the cup of quinoa and of simply boil water (10 fl oz - 300ml).

3. Diminish the heat to a stew, place the top on and permit to cook. Throughout the following 30 minutes, blending at regular intervals or so to ensure nothing adheres to the base. As it cooks, include the chickpeas.

4. When there are only 5 minutes left, include the spinach and mix it in until it withers. After the quinoa has cooked and is cushioned, not crunchy, it's prepared.

5. On the off chance that you like a touch of heat, add a cut red bean stew to the cooking curry simultaneously as different flavors

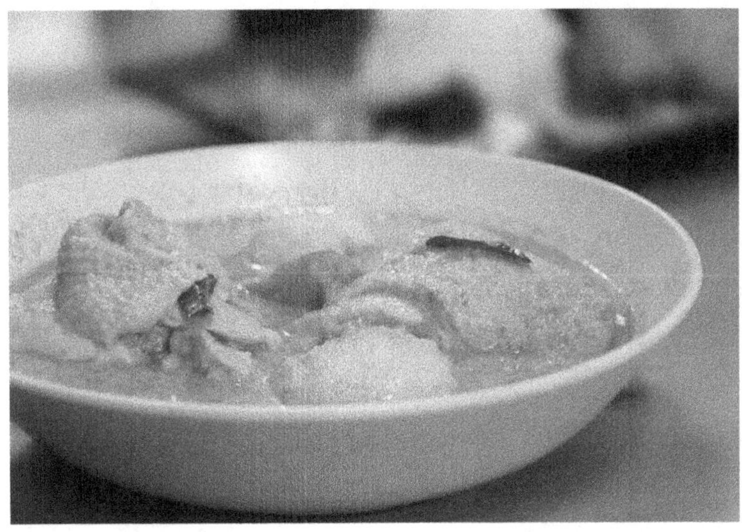

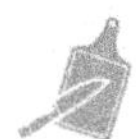 **15 mins** 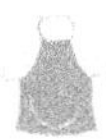 **40 mins** 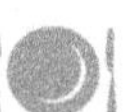 1 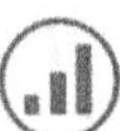 Calories: 345 - Fat: 9.5g – Fiber: 12g
Carbs: 65.76g - Protein: 12.5g

COD MARINATED IN MISO

Ingredients:

- ½ oz (15 g) miso
- ½ fl oz (30 ml) Chinese wine
- ½ fl oz (30 ml) olive oil
- 7 ⅔ oz (220 g) cod fillet
- ½ oz (15 g) white onion, chopped
- 1 oz (30 g) celery stalk
- 1 garlic, minced
- 1 pc bird's eye chili, finely chopped
- 1 tsp ginger powder
- 2 ⅓ oz (65 g) green beans
- 2 oz (60 g) Kale, strips
- ½ tsp sesame seeds
- ⅓ oz (10 g) parsley
- ½ fl oz (30 ml) light soy sauce
- 1½ oz (40 g) buckwheat
- 1 tsp turmeric

Directions:

1. Combine the Chinese wine, miso, and oil in a bowl. Put cod and soak it to marinate. Chill for about 30 minutes. Preheat the oven at 200c.
2. After the cod marinates, put the cod in the baking pan and let it bake for 10-15 Minutes.
3. In a separate pan, heat oil and add all ingredients except buckwheat, turmeric, tamari, sesame seeds and tamari. Stir-fry and don't overcook
4. Cook the buckwheat with turmeric.
5. After cooking, add parsley, sesame seeds and tamari.
6. Stir-fry then serve with the cod and greens.

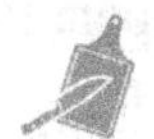 **5 mins**  **10 mins**  1

Calories: 360 - Fat: 10g – Fiber: 11.5g
Carbs: 64.8g - Protein: 13.2g

Ingredients:

- 3½ oz (100 g) raspberries washed
- 2 pcs gelatin leaves

- 3½ oz (100 g) blackcurrants
- 1 fl oz (30 ml) white sugar
- 10 fl oz (300 ml) water

Directions:

1. Put the raspberries into a mold or glass. In a bowl of cold water, bloom gelatin leaves until soft.
2. Put the blackcurrants in a pot with sugar and water, then bring to a boil. As it reaches boiling point, lower it down to simmering heat and let cook for five minutes.
3. Turn off the heat and let it cool down for 2 minutes. Take the gelatin leaves out from the first bowl and squeeze out the water.
4. Add it to the pan and mix well.
5. Pour the whole mixture into the mold and chill until it becomes jelly. It may take about 3-4 hrs. Or you can wait overnight too.

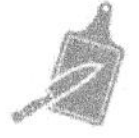 3/4 hrs. 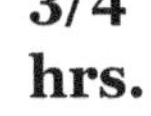 10 mins 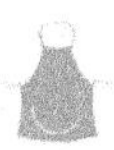 1 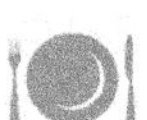

Calories: 15 - Fat: 4.3g – Fiber: 1.4g
Carbs: 34g - Protein: 1.4g

Ingredients:

- 2 pcs Bosc pears
- ¼ cup Cherries, pitted
- 8 fl oz (250 ml) Red wine
- 2 fl oz (60 ml) Orange juice
- 1 pc Cloves
- ½ tsp Vanilla extract
- 2 tbsp Date sugar
- 1 pc Cinnamon stick
- Orange zest

Directions:

1. Add all of your red wine poached pear ingredients, except for the Bosc pears, into a large Dutch oven. You need a pot large enough to fit all six whole hears. You want them to fit snugly so that the pears are fully covered in the liquid, but still have a slight wiggle room. But, remember, don't add the pears yet.

2. Allow the wine mixture to reach a simmer in the pot while stirring to dissolve the date sugar.

3. Wait until the poaching liquid has reached a simmer and then peel the pears. This will help avoid discoloration. Place the pears into the poaching liquid, arranging them so that they are submerged.

4. Allow the pears to continue simmering on medium-low for about twenty to twenty-five minutes. But while the pears poach rearrange and rotate them every five minutes. Don't skip this, as it will ensure they poach evenly on all sides. You want to ensure even the tops of the pears are well poached.

5. Once the pears are done poaching, keep the pears upright in the wine mixture. Remove the pot from the heat of the stove, and allow both the pears and poaching liquid to cool down together.

6. While you can serve the poached pears once cooled to room temperature, I recommend first chilling them in the fridge.

7. When chilling the pears in the fridge, keep them stored in the liquid.

8. Once you are ready to serve the pears, remove them from the liquid and set them on serving dishes. Meanwhile, add the poaching liquid into a saucepan and allow it to simmer to heat until it forms a slightly thickened syrup.

9. Pour the red wine syrup over the cold pears and serve.

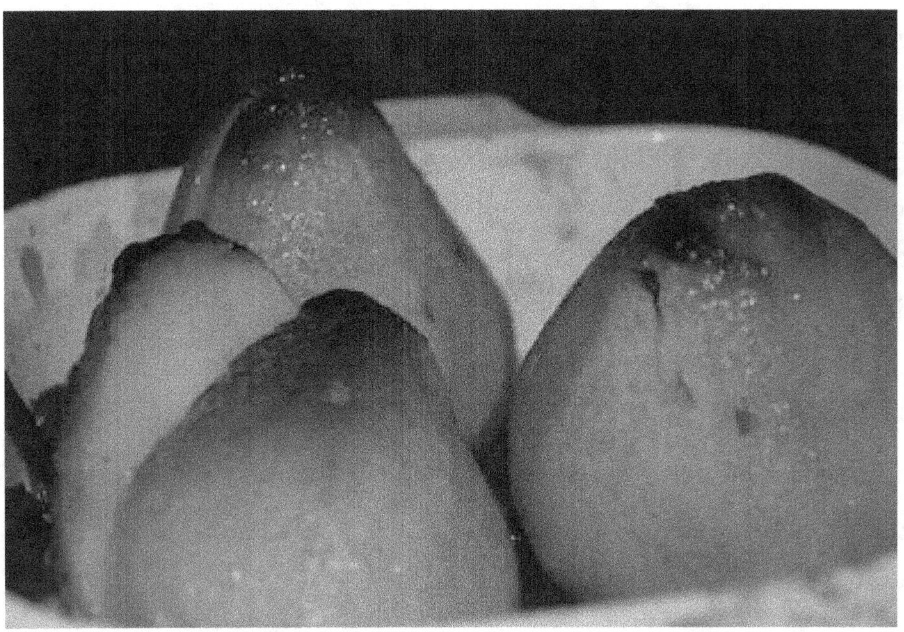

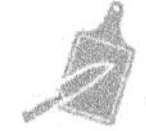 **15/30 mins.** 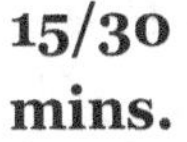 **30 mins**  1  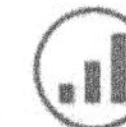 Calories: 298 - Fat: 2.4g – Fiber: 7.6g
Carbs: 45.8g - Protein: 3.1g

Chapter 14

Sirtfood and Exercise

The combination of exercise with a balanced diet is one successful method in losing weight than relying solely on calorie limits. Exercise can avoid the symptoms of such diseases, or even reverse them. Exercise can lower cholesterol and blood pressure, thereby avoiding a heart attack.

Additionally, you lower chance the development of definite types of cancers such as breast cancer and colon cancer if you have exercise activities. Exercise is recognized to help lead to a sense of confidence and wellbeing, potentially reducing levels of depression and anxiety.

Exercising is useful for losing weight and gaining weight. Exercise will improve metabolism as well as adjust the calories you consume in one day. It will also help in maintaining and increasing lean body mass, which also helps to increase the calories you utilize every day.

To enjoy the health benefits of exercise, it is encouraged that you do some type of aerobic exercise for at least 20 minutes per day, at least three days a week. Over 20 minutes, though, is better if you actually want to lose weight. Incorporating only 20 minutes of exercise — like walking one mile — on a regular basis, will burn up to 80 extra calories. Being able to burn 700 calories per week can amount to 10 lbs. of weight loss in one year.

To maintain physical and mental health and wellbeing, it is important to eat a healthy balanced diet followed by exercising regularly. These do not only have an effective result in preventing excess weight gain or in holding weight loss but also associate healthy lifestyles with better mood and sleep Physical activity significantly gives improvement function and outcomes related to the brain.

The Sirtfood Diet is designed to help you activate your sirtuin genes without the necessity of exercise or fasting, but that doesn't mean you shouldn't add regular and consistent physical activity to your life to protect your body from deterioration and aging in other ways.

Your nutrition can do the lion's share of maintaining health and preventing disease, but if you don't use your body and muscles on a regular basis, they will atrophy, stiffen up and stop working for you.

What this means primarily is that exercise doesn't have to be your go-to solution for weight loss or weight management. Still, rather it should be practiced as a means of maintaining our ability to move and stay strong and energetic.

Our bodies were designed to go through a wide range of movements, from the bending, pulling, and lifting required to farm, gather and harvest, to the cardiovascular capacity to hunt and the combination of all of the above that is required to keep children occupied and safe.

In short, even if a Sirtfood Diet helps you fight disease and reach your ideal body weight, you shouldn't neglect your exercise.

Muscle and Strength

When you're completely sedentary, doing nothing but lounging in front of your television or working at a computer desk, your muscles require about 30% of the energy your body needs to keep you just sitting there.

When you exercise, your muscles use closer to 90% of your energy. As you can imagine, this will burn up a lot more carbohydrates and fat than simply sitting in your chair, but you knew that already.

The less you use your muscles, the smaller and weaker they will get, but again, this is not news.

Why is muscle mass and strength so important to our health?

One reason is that studies show that, of all causes of mortality, the risk of death for individuals classified as "strong" is about half that of those classified as "weak." The stronger you are, the more likely you are to stay alive simply. That is certainly motivating.

Approximately 60% of Americans have at least one chronic disease. That number increases to more than 90% when the population is limited to adults over 65 years of age.

65 is not old, and we should all be expecting to live at least that long, and many of us much longer. But 65 years of inactivity is a long time to allow your muscles to shrink, and this is a major contributing factor to the prevalence of chronic diseases at this age.

One particularly shocking disease is sarcopenia, the age-related wasting of our muscles. As we age, we naturally start to lose muscle mass and strength at a rate of about 3% or more per decade after we reach our 30s. This is in addition to the muscle we lose simply from being sedentary. That muscle is usually traded in for fat.

Muscle mass is not purely designed for aesthetic purposes. It is associated with both our balance and our bone density, which can lead to frailty and loss of independence in our future.

But it isn't just in our retirement years that a lack of muscle will start to really affect us. Diseases such as cancer, renal failure, heart disease, and rheumatoid and osteoarthritis are all linked to lower muscle mass, both as a cause and as a result.

We know sirtfoods can help protect our muscle mass, but how should we build it?
Exercise during the initial barely any weeks

During the main week or two of the diet where your calorie admission is diminished, it is reasonable to stop or lessen practice while your body adjusts to fewer calories. Tune in to your body, and if you feel exhausted or have less vitality than expected, don't work out. Rather guarantee that you stay concentrated on the rules that apply to a solid lifestyle, for example, including satisfactory day by day levels of fiber, protein, and products of the soil.

In the first phase of the Sirtfood Diet or any time in your life that you're reducing calories for any other reason, the moderate movement suggestions. But to live a full, healthy, and strong life, we will need to dedicate more energy specifically toward our muscles.

Our bodies are designed to adapt to what becomes a normal movement. If you've never gone for a jog before in your life, the first block is going to be a struggle. But if you practice every day, your body adapts, and jogging 1 block will become easy.

If you have never lifted a baby before and you find yourself having to carry one around for 8 -10 hours a day, even a tiny 7-pound newborn is going to feel heavy at first. But after a few weeks of parenthood, your body will adapt, you will become stronger, and even when your baby weighs 20 pounds, you won't find them too heavy to manage.

We are not all going to be carrying around growing babies all our lives; however, so a smart way to grow your muscles using the same principle is to either lift weights or use your bodyweight.

Using weights gives you the ability to track any improvements in strength as you find yourself progressively adding more weight to your lifting. However, bodyweight exercises have the distinct advantage of not requiring any equipment, and they use dynamic movements, which also help to improve total body wellness, flexibility, and mobility.

Bodyweight exercises include movements like pushups, pullups, squats, and lunges, taking the stairs, and even holding many yoga poses.

You don't have to give your entire life over to becoming an athlete. You can see dramatic results in as little as 3 days a week, only 30 minutes at a time.

If you begin progressively building strength from a younger age, you will protect yourself against many so-called chronic and age-related diseases. If you are already in the range of 65+ years of age, all is not lost.

With the permission and guidance of your doctor, if you begin challenging your muscles now, you can build them up again and begin to recover from any diseases related to muscle loss that you may already have. You will have to begin slowly and carefully, but the results can change your outlook on life quickly within just a few weeks of training.

A Sirtfood diet will help to protect the muscle you have. Still, to really combat this natural process, you should be dedicated to actively strengthening your muscles throughout your entire life. Lifting weights or doing progressively more challenging bodyweight exercises is a great way to build your muscles.

Summary & Key Takeaways

In our youth, we may take the ability to move our body for granted, but if you neglect physical exercise for too many years, your body will lose its ability to move, no matter how many sirtfoods you're eating.

Exercise doesn't have to be a painful experience requiring you to spend hours a week at the gym, lifting heavy weights and running miles on a treadmill. It's far more effective to move your body in a way that you would like to continue to be able to move your body.

Imagine yourself at 60 or 80 or 100 years old. What types of activities would you love to be still able to do? Most of us don't expect to be joining sports leagues or beating our personal best records at this age, but if we live that long, we do want to be able to enjoy it.

Small things, like being able to sit on the floor playing with your great-great-grandchildren and then be able to stand up again without assistance. Or perhaps be able to carry our own groceries into the house. Dancing at a family member's wedding, or going fishing. Whatever your personal goals are for your future, you have to create muscle memory to ensure your body will be able to continue to support the type of movement you want to participate in.

Participating in regular physical activity protects your bones and your joints, and promotes effective blood circulation as well. It has been proven to reduce stress and improve mental health. Sirtfoods can help with all of these areas of your life, but when you're talking about your health, it's best to incorporate as many positive factors as possible.

As a society, we've adjusted to accepting normal or average as the most we expect to get out of life when, in truth, with a little added effort, we can go well beyond average. Men in Sardinia, Italy, are hiking up mountains to harvest honey at 100+ years old, and the women of Ikaria, Greece, are preparing fresh pasta for their 4th and 5th generation grandchildren every week. Surely, we can raise the bar for ourselves as well.

Chapter 15

Types of Exercise You Can Do

Rules to Keep in Mind

- Before you do any type of physical activity, it is better to take an examination that will let you know if you are capable of dotting it or what restrictions must be set.

- Try to stay away from activities with a big impact on joints. Which can cause the joints excessively?

- You prefer sports such as cycling, swimming, or walking. Sports that require certain steps of graduality are the only ones capable of counteracting osteoporosis and of promoting calcium metabolism

- Do aerobic activity. It begins gradually with sessions under 10 minutes, intermixed with short breaks. Incrementally for 20, 30 minutes.

- Do stretching exercises, in moderation, to make you more flexible.

- Do not train during the hottest hours of the day in summer or in too cold or humid environments in winter.

- Consume 2 liters of water or more days and during training, with frequent small sips.

- Choose surfaces that are flat for jogging, with the right type of shoes to avoid muscle pain or inflammation.

- Don't put a limitation on just sitting in the gym or your daily sports minutes. Grab every chance you get to move.

Tone the Lean Mass

It is wrong to be focusing only on aerobic exercises, forgetting the toning and anaerobic aspect. Spending a lot of hours on a treadmill certainly promotes fat consumption. But excessive fat loss predisposes our body to the release of the stress hormone, cortisol. It will lower down the rate of metabolism, will be accelerating water retention and having the feeling of general tiredness. Indeed, when one feels too tired and the body will be less toned.

A correct training card must take into account the basic muscle composition, for women in particular, of the targeted training needs for legs, buttocks and abdominals, to ensure good toning for a pleasant aesthetic.

At the level of muscle growth, men and women share the same structure. The obvious difference lies in the production of natural testosterone, which obviously is higher in men and allows them to increase mass in a much more important way.

To obtain the desired results, therefore, we must integrate training with exercises that use weights and machines. Strength training, with weights, barbells and kettlebells, studied on individual needs, is the right way to tone your muscles.

Power-ups with tools are important for developing lean mass over fat. The calorie expenditure associated with tonic muscles is higher than the fat mass. It is possible to eat the same, following a sirt diet but consuming more calories per day. Muscle development and endurance allow bones to remain compact, useful for preventing osteoporosis.

High-Intensity Interval Training (HIIT)

Recent studies have shown that to combat disease, one of the most effective ways to exercise is to combine strength training with aerobic and endurance exercise.

High-intensity interval training, or HIIT, does just that. This type of exercise combines anaerobic movements designed to improve strength and power in short bursts of intense effort with recovery periods.

Depending on the specific program, the usual routine requires all of your energy for only 10 – 30 seconds at a time, followed by a rest or recovery period of up to 1.5 minutes. This movement or a combination of exercises is repeated 5 to 10 times, so you end up devoting a maximum of 20 minutes to this type of program.

This rapid cycling of intense movements activates "fast-twitch muscle fibers." We all have 2 different types of muscles in our body: slow-twitch muscle is designed to support us through long durations of moderate activity, whereas fast-twitch muscles power us through short bursts of intense activity.

Interestingly, the way we eat also impacts these two different types of muscles. Fasting is another way to activate sirtuins. When you fast as a way to lose weight or improve your health metrics, your sirtuins effectively protect your slow-twitch muscle fibers and may even help them grow, but your fast-twitch muscle fibers actually decline rapidly. If you activate your sirtuins through the addition of sirtfoods, fast-twitch muscle fibers actually increase in size. This makes the Sirtfood Diet a great complement to the occasional HIIT workout.

Studies show that when you participate in high-intensity training, you not only burn through the sugars that are freely flowing through your bloodstream, but your body will also tap into the fat stores that you're trying to reduce as a way to fuel your body through the short-term acute stress of this type of workout.

By doing so, you'll be able to improve your metabolic and hormonal functioning, including insulin and leptin resistance, at the same time as you build muscles, improve the health of your heart and increase your cardiorespiratory endurance as well.

In other parts, we've talked a little bit about your mitochondria, the powerhouse of your cells that converts incoming glucose to the energy your body uses to operate. HIIT has been shown to improve the export of energy from your mitochondria in order to meet the demands of intense physical activity.

By upgrading their capacity, you're not only keeping your cells in healthy working order, but you're also increasing the availability of energy to provide to your muscles, improving your performance and endurance. It is a very powerful cycle that essentially compounds the benefits to your body over time.

The Sirtfood Diet gained a lot of popularity through celebrity culture and, particularly, the fact this it is a diet that many athletes have adopted to keep them lean and strong at the same time, including rugby stars and Olympic gold medalists among others. They may not know all practice HIIT, but it cannot be argued that an elite athlete has a highly intensive workout regimen.

Fitness for Women

Women choose fitness to keep fit, to lose a few extra pounds and, more and more frequently, to feel good about themselves. Taking care of your body's health with sport is not easy. So much so that you can run into many mistakes. One of the most common mistakes is to avoid warming up before starting training.

This practice is very important because it allows the body to enter the temperature. For toned abs, it is enough to dedicate yourself as for the other muscles, two or three times a week, with a couple of sets done carefully and slowly. It is not advisable to practice long series of exercises. Otherwise, the result could be a prominent abdomen and possible damage to the back and posture

To obtain a harmonic body, we must not underestimate any part of our body. Stretch and squat push-ups and assume fundamental importance for the toning of all parts of the body. Push-ups, in particular, represent one of the few exercises that, in one gesture, set muscles in the whole body in motion.

The endorphins, after a training session, make us feel exhausted but enthusiastic, to the point that we can't wait to go back to the gym. In doing so, there is a risk of straining the muscle with harmful injuries

Rest, in fact, is as important as training. It is good to give a certain muscle band a break of at least 48.

Breathing is important, like rest, if you want to maximize the effectiveness of training. Constancy is the key to obtaining the desired results thanks to sports and fitness. The ideal would soon be to find a balance that allows you to combine family, work, commitments and training. The goal can only be achieved if this is sustainable in the long run.

Targeted Exercises

Training in the wrong way has as a first effect on not being able to achieve the goals we have set. If we desire our body to have more harmony, toned, and lean, and we don't expect the right rules, we probably won't see the change we want.

A wrong method, excessive training intensity, a concentrated effort on some muscles or limbs make the chances of obtaining microtraumas or other injuries higher. Training will soon become a source of stress and frustration, if we do not take note of our mistakes, with the only result of letting us abandon our program.

It is easy to get caught up in enthusiasm and choose to train to start from easy exercises setting your own goals, which are, of course, subjective and personal.

Aerobic activities stimulate the body to use large quantities of oxygen and help the muscles and encourage the consumption of calories.

For women who aspire to have a harmonious body and want to tone their body, it would be advisable to practice a complete workout, even at the time of music, which includes push-ups, bends, stretches, and exercises with small dumbbells and kettlebells.

Various Exercises

To work completely on the whole musculature, with harmonious effects on an aesthetic level and health benefits, a weekly training session for women, must take into account the variability of the weights and the intensity of the training.

Contrary to what many women think, it will not be some exercise commensurate with their body to disfigure the female body with man exercises. In any case, weight training is essential, alternating with aerobics. The equipment will be suitable for those who use them are beginners or habitual to these practices.

Below is an example of a program that requires continuous work in order to burn the largest number of energies. Obviously, it is enough to choose only one activity per session.

- treadmill for cardio exercise - 10 minutes
- oblique crunch for abs - 3 sets x 12 reps per side
- crunch on the flat bench for abs - 3 sets x 15 reps
- pelvis twists - 3 sets x max repetitions in 1 minute
- adductor machine for inner thigh - 3 sets x 15 reps
- abductor machine for external thigh - 3 sets x 15 reps
- leg press for legs - 3 sets x 12 reps
- step for cardio exercise - 15 minutes
- elliptical trainer for cardio exercise - 10 minutes
- presses on an inclined bench for the chest - 3 sets for 15 repetitions

- triceps with a dumbbell behind - 3 sets for 12 reps
- lat machine ahead for the backbones - 3 sets for 12 reps
- exercise bike for cardio exercise - 5 minutes

Program why you want to work on gaining muscle mass, using bodybuilding machines. You can start using light loads.

- treadmill or stepper or elliptical - 10 minutes
- abdominal machine for the abdominals - 25 kg of weight for 2 sets and 10 reps (to be increased up to 35 kg of weight for 3 sets with 15 reps)
- abdominal crunch - 2 sets for 12 reps

Leg press for legs - 40 kg weight for 2 sets and 10 reps (to be increased up to 55 kg for 3 sets and 12 reps)

- gluteus machine for the buttocks - 10 kg of weight for 2 sets and 10 reps (to be increased up to 25 kg for 3 sets and 15 reps)
- adductor machine for inner thigh - 15 kg of weight for 2 sets and 12 reps (to be increased up to 55 kg for 3 sets and 15 reps)
- shoulder press for shoulders - 10 kg of weight for 2 sets and 10 reps (to be increased up to 15 kg for 3 sets and 12 reps)
- triceps at the top cables - 10 kg weight for 2 sets and 10 repetitions (to be increased up to 20 kg for 3 sets and 12 repetitions)
- chest press for the chest - 10 kg of weight for 2 sets and 10 reps (to be increased up to 25 kg for 3 sets and 15 reps)

Back pulley - 10 kg weight for 2 sets and 10 reps (to be increased up to 15 kg for 3 sets and 15 reps)

- treadmill - 5 minutes.

This training of about 3 sessions per week will be ideal if the training is carried out constantly and gradually.

Chapter 16

A Health-Focused Diet Plan for Life

We hopefully have given you all the motivation and determination you need to not just make it through the first 2 phases of a Sirtfood Diet, but to continue incorporating sirtfoods into your meals for the rest of your life.

There may come times when you feel like you need a reboot, and when or if that happens, you can repeat the first or second phase as needed. But if you make nutrient-dense, health-focused eating your new way of life, you will continue to see the unnecessary weight melt off of you and unwelcome signs of ill health plague you less and less frequently.

From now on, you will have more energy powering you through your day than you ever realized was even possible. You'll be sleeping more deeply, laughing more frequently, and spending much more time enjoying everything life has to offer, including delicious meals.

The Sirtfood Diet was never meant to be a quick fix or to last only for 3 weeks. It is a lifestyle.

Never Diet Again

Perhaps the greatest thing about the Sirtfood Diet is the fact that if you incorporate these foods into your life on a daily basis, you will find that you never have to even think about dieting again. You will attain your goal weight with patience and dedication, and it won't come back.

Not only will you be at your ideal body weight, but you'll have more energy, clearer skin, a healthier heart, and a stronger body, and you'll be happier than you can remember ever being. Such is the power of sirtuin-activating foods.

You will notice that the more you eat the nutrient-dense plants that are encouraged in the Sirtfood Diet, and drink your concentrated shot of sirtuin-activating compounds in your green juice, the more your body and taste buds are going to demand you continue blessing them with such great fuel. Before you even realize it, you will see a bag of chips or a doughnut that would have made you drool in longing just a few weeks or months ago, and the thought of eating it will turn your stomach.

There will be a learning curve as you get used to swapping out low-quality food options for nutrient-dense choices. But if you make it easy for yourself to make these choices, they will become automatic much quicker than you would believe possible.

When you're shopping for your groceries, buy buckwheat pasta and whole-grain bread. Have a selection of fresh herbs, sweet and tart berries, nuts and seeds on hand to sprinkle over top of every meal. Stop buying soda and start experimenting with the different roasts of coffee, varieties of tea, and, in moderation, blends of red wine.

Challenge yourself and your family members to try a new plant-based item each week, or find new ways to use the ingredients you're already comfortable with. Everything about food should be an enjoyable event, from the choosing of the highest quality ingredients to cooking with love and eating with joy. Best of all, after every meal, you won't be suffering from nagging feelings of guilt and heartburn, but instead, you'll be invigorated and proud of yourself.

There will likely be times in your life where your diet goes astray. Perhaps you go on vacation, or you get injured and can't cook as much as you would like to. Maybe it's the holiday season, and the power of comfort foods and nostalgic cooking overwhelmed you. Whatever the reason, acknowledge that you're human, and a setback doesn't have to hold you back or completely derail all your hard work.

If you feel like you could benefit from another reset, you can repeat Stage 1 and Stage 2 of the Sirtfood diet for a refresher and a boost to your life-long commitment to health. Many people around the world regularly fast for a few weeks or even a month a year with no caloric intake at all. Stage 1 is simply a modest reduction in calories, and it can do a lot of good for your mindset.

Taking any portion of this diet and using it to excuse or counteract poor eating habits is not only advised, nor is it ideal for your health. Any type of caloric restriction should be limited to only a short period of time, and adding sirtfoods to your meals should be done as consistently as possible. There is no good excuse for abusing your health, even if you think your sirtuin genes will be there to save the day.

Stage 2 doesn't require any calorie restriction, so it can be repeated as often as you'd like. Some people prefer the structure of the maintenance phase and continue eating this way indefinitely. It was designed to create a balanced, life-long blueprint for creating your eating patterns, and if continuing this phase helps you to stick to your commitment, it will only be to the benefit of your health.

Embrace a Diet of Inclusion

A very common by-product of a poor diet is a very broken relationship with the food we eat. As a society, most of us have become very removed from the source of our food. We actively avoid learning where the animal products are coming from or how they were produced, and many children are growing up unable to identify freshly harvested fruits and vegetables. They may know that carrots are orange, but they've only ever seen them cubed in pre-packed frozen or canned foods.

Because of this distance, we have lost respect for the food we're eating. For most of us, it's readily available whenever we want it, so we take it for granted. This often encourages us to overconsume, especially if we also factor in the additives that are in pre-made foods.

When we eat food that doesn't nourish us, our bodies rebel, we feel sick, tired, and unhappy. So we start to tell ourselves all the things we're not allowed to do. We can't eat our favorite cookies, and we're no longer allowed to go out for our favorite fast food. We can't have more than 800 calories a day, and we can't eat any carbs/fat/sugar, etc.

All of this pressure makes us feel guilty about every morsel of food we eat, but we're so deeply engrained in the cycle that it's very difficult to tunnel our ways out without help.

The Sirtfood Diet is your help. It is your guide back to real, whole, and nourishing foods. While you are encouraged to trade in the foods that are well known to damage your health, the focus isn't on what you can't have. The focus of the Sirtfood Diet is welcoming in an entire category of foods that you can have, in almost unlimited supply.

The concept of calculating calories is new, as far as human evolution is concerned. Traditional societies don't restrict what they're eating based on a label that tells them what the net carbs of their food are. The healthiest cultures in the world consume food that doesn't come with labels. It comes out of the ground, is husbanded on a farm, or fished out of the sea. They eat the food that they naturally have access to, appreciate and respect their value, and stop eating when they're full.

When you're first getting started, you might want to limit your exciting new food adventures to familiarizing yourself closely with the top 20 sirtfoods. They are going to give you the most instant success and power you through the first few weeks of a new eating plan.

As you grow comfortable with these ingredients, you can start to experiment with other plant-based, polyphenol-rich foods. There are more edible plants in the world than you will probably ever have the opportunity to try, so adding one or two to your repertoire each week will ensure that you're always trying something new and giving yourself permission to include more and more foods into your diet.

There will be no guilt when you eat nourishing foods. The only thing you will be saying no to is ill health. When you open up to the possibility of eating everything that can improve your health, your options expand well beyond what you're used to. The Sirtfood Diet is founded on diversity and inclusion. The more nutrients, the merrier!

Sustaining Lifestyle Changes and Choices

Devoting yourself to being mindful of your food choices isn't the only other change you will have to sustain in your life if you truly want to be committed to retaining your health and maintaining healthy body weight.

You were encouraged to let go of target weight goals and instead replace them with health goals. Good health is a lifetime achievement, with no end date. Chances are, you still kept a magic number in your mind as you kept reading this. When you start the first 2 stages of the diet, hopefully, you'll see enough positive changes to refocus your attention on health and away from the weight aspect. If you stick to the Sirtfood Diet, however, there will come a day when you realized you'd reached that magic number.

When that happens, you should celebrate your accomplishments. Having healthy body composition is an incredible indicator of health, and its something to be very proud of. But don't let this achievement affect your future success. You certainly don't have to restrict calories anymore and possibly never again. Still, if you want to stay healthy, you do need to continue feeding your body all the nourishment it has come to know, love, and deserves. Sirtfoods are a part of your life now and forever.

As we talked about, you also need to make physical movement a lifestyle choice, not a temporary fix. Exercise is just as important to your long-term health as the right nutrition plan is, and the need for physical movement doesn't disappear just because you can fit into your skinny jeans again. To stay strong, fit and healthy, you need to stay active.

One of the most effective ways to make the changes you're now making last a lifetime is to turn them into habitual behaviors. The only secret to making healthy habits stick is repetition over time. All you need is dedication upfront, and you'll reap the rewards without a second thought for the rest of your life.

Think about some of the actions that have been a part of your life for a long time. You probably have a well-established routine that you don't put any thought into, you simply act. For example, maybe in the morning, you get up, shower, have a coffee and maybe some breakfast, and then drive to the office. You're there before you realize it, and then you go through the motions of your job. This routine has become a habit for you. It's not hard to do, and it's just something you do.

To help yourself turn your healthy choices into sustainable life-long habits, try incorporating them into your life on a set schedule or routine. Drink your green juices at the same time each day. Eat your meals at the same time each day.

Do your shopping and meal prepping and batch cooking on the same days each week. Schedule in specific activities on a regular basis to stay active. Your body will come to expect these actions, and before you know it, you will begin craving a green juice in the morning. You'll find the time you spend in your kitchen more relaxing and cathartic, and you'll look forward to seeing what new strengths and abilities your body has advanced to with each scheduled exercise program.

As your routines and habits develop over time, you won't just be following the Sirtfood Diet for your health, and you'll be following it because you enjoy it and look forward to each day.

Chapter 17

Tips and Advice

Obviously, even if up to now we have enhanced the properties of sirtuins and the Sirt diet, to obtain better results in terms of weight loss and health, it is also necessary to adopt a correct lifestyle and virtuous habits. The general rules of a healthy lifestyle are very easy to follow and applied every day. From eating nutritious food to exercising, here's how to behave to live long and healthy.

The essential aspects of a healthy lifestyle, which leaves you feeling good for a long time are within everyone's capability, even if we often forget about it.

- Drink about two liters of plain water per day

- Eat lots of seasonal fruit and vegetables

- Moderate fats, especially saturated ones

- Moderate your sugar intake

- Moderate salt consumption

- Don't smoke

- Keep Moving!

- Get enough sleep

- Don't skip meals! Fasting does not help you lose weight quickly ...

- Review your eating habits

- Brush your teeth after eating!

- Drink tea and herbal teas to lose weight quickly

- Do your shopping on a full stomach

Hacking the Skinny Genes

Genes contain data that determine everything from appearance to intelligence. An individual acquires genes from their parents, and how parents live affects their offspring's' genes.

It's a mixed-up supposition that all that you acquired in your genes is changeless. Your way of life and conditions can stir single genes or potentially smother others. Here are ways you can modify your condition and way of life to improve your body and brain.

1. Your health will depend on the type of food you eat.
Food and nutrients are significant - both can impact the body and psyche. On the off chance that you consistently eat solid and nutritious food, your genes will react as needs to be. Sound sustenance stirs essential genes that positively affect your brain and body. It's basic to have a reliably sound diet since you need your great genes to be dynamic.

Keep up a truly thorough food plan consistently. Your food plan might comprise a free form of the paleo diet. In addition to the fact that this keeps will keep the brain sharp, yet it encourages and keeps up an optimal execution when working out. Try not to take alcohol, don't smoke and don't do any form of drugs. You feel healthier than you will ever be.

2. Stress can initiate changes.
Everyone manages pressure, and that can affect our health and genes. In case you're reliably worried, certain valuable genes can progressively get smothered or enacted to enable you to adapt. That can directly affect your efficiency and health.

To battle pressure, you can go on long runs or drive while tuning in to your preferred music. Utilize positive mental quality tricks and breathing activities to help still your mind and slow your pulse down.

3. A functioning way of life will stir the best genes.

A functioning way of life impacts changes also. You don't need to be an activity addict to get great outcomes. You should simply enjoy some physical movement, for example, moving or running all the time. Your body will initiate genes expected to help those exercises after some time. The effect has a net positive on your health, mind, and profitability.

4. Change your condition.

Once in a while, changing your condition isn't as simple as affecting different parts of your life. However, you can control it in little manners. Normal introduction to morning daylight, a clean home environment, and living close to a green zone can impact your dynamic genes, mind, body, and even your state of mind.

You are keeping the entirety of the workplace clean and mess-free. You should continually change where you work and travel. For me, the result is a substantially more productive, unique way of life.

Tips Before, During and After Diet

Even though the first period of the Sirtfood Diet is deficient in calories and healthfully fragmented, there are no genuine security worries for the healthy, sound grown-up thinking about the eating regimen's brief span.

However, for somebody with diabetes, calorie limitation and drinking for the most part squeeze for the initial scarcely any days of the eating regimen may cause risky changes in glucose levels

In any case, even a stable individual may encounter some reactions — basically hunger. Eating just 1,000–1,500 calories for every day will leave pretty much anybody feeling hungry, mainly if quite a bit of what you're expending is juice, which is low in fiber, a supplement that helps keep you feeling full

During phase one, you may encounter different symptoms, for example, weakness, tipsiness, and touchiness because of the calorie limitation. For the, in any case, dependable grown-up, positive wellbeing results are far-fetched if the eating regimen is followed for just three weeks. Being a calorie-restricted diet, mainly phase one in the Sirt food diet, isn't healthfully adjusted. It might leave you hungry. However, it's not dangerous for the average sound grown-up.

Taking a gander at the rundown of nutrients, you can see they are the kind of things that frequently show up on a 'sound food list,' anyway it is smarter to energize these as a significant aspect of a solid adjusted eating regimen.

Having a glass of red wine or a modest quantity of chocolate once in a while won't do us any mischief anyway. It isn't prescribed to follow consistently. We ought to likewise be eating a blend of various foods grown from the ground and not only those on the rundown.

As far as weight reduction and boosting digestion, individuals may have encountered a seven-pound weight reduction on the scales, yet I would say this will be liquid. Consuming and losing fat requires some investment.

When individuals come back to their habitual dietary patterns, they will recover the weight. Gradual weight reduction is the key, and for this, we have to limit calories and increment our activity levels.

Gobbling adjusted standard suppers comprised of low GI nutrients, lean protein, foods grown from the ground, and keeping all-around hydrated is the most secure approach to get in shape. Follow the following pieces of advice to be more successful:

Be kind to yourself - Do not set too high expectations. Yes, some can easily lose 7 pounds in a week, but remember that our bodies are not all the same; and of course, your level of commitment will also count. Other variables could be adding an exercise regimen in the diet plan, which could make the losing weight process faster.

Plan your meals ahead - Whatever diet you may be on, planning your meals is a big help. Not only will it reduce the stress from dieting, but you can also have the chance to weigh your choices and fill in your cupboard. For the first phase of this diet, you have to follow a calorie count. You will be surprised that there are many filling dishes allowed with fewer calories and packed with sirtuins.

Hit the supermarket - The SirtFood diet depends on certain foods. These foods were chosen because of their sirtuin-triggering ability. So, if you do not follow the list, well, you won't see results. Do not worry, because I will be providing the list of suggested foods; Plus, there is no overly expensive type of foods, and you can find it readily available almost anywhere (you might even already have some lurking in your fridge).

Follow the guidelines - SirtFood is guaranteed to bring results, if and only if you carefully follow the diet guide and suggested food.

Help yourself - Aside from following what is allowed in the food program, and you can start by eliminating processed and starchy food from your normal diet. Stop eating junk! This will fast track the result of SirtFood Diet.

Chapter 18

Frequently Asked Questions

Is it OK to exercise during phase 1 of the program?

Nothing wrong can come if you exercise during this phase of the sirtfood diet. Moderate exercise is highly recommended, but if you choose to go for intense training, keep in mind that this will use up your energy reserves (most likely). If you are used to a moderate level of training, then the best way is to continue the same level during the first phase of this program. Intense exercise can do the fat burning for you, but it can also make your feed again, although you shouldn't have to. Therefore, keep it moderate and let the sirtfood diet do the work for you.

What's the purpose of following this diet if I'm already slim?

The first phase of the sirtfood diet should not be tried by underweight people. How can you tell if you are underweight? Just check your body mass index (BMI) level. Any person with a BMI below 18.5 is considered underweight, so phase 1 of this program should not be tried by them. Keep in mind that the maintenance phase can also lead to fat loss, but it can help you build muscle as well. The underweight people should benefit from the activation of sirtuins, but they need to consume a lot less amount of food compared to overweight people.

Is the sirtfood diet right for me if I'm obese?

Although a small number of participants in the pilot study were obese, I can only encourage obese people to try this diet in the long term. Why? Because it creates the perfect environment in your body to lose weight. Obese people need to lose weight constantly in the long run, not to lose a lot of weight dramatically in a very short amount of time. If this diet worked for people and they lost seven pounds in seven days, this rate could be considered satisfactory for them. However, they need to alternate the first phase and the second phase.

I managed to reach the weight I want, and I simply don't want to lose any more weight. Do I have to stop eating sirtfoods?

Achieving your objectives can only prove that this diet works. So the first phase worked like a charm for you. Even though you don't want to lose any more weight, you can stick to the maintenance phase for a long time. You have to benefit from sirtuins for life. After all, this diet is also about health benefits, and if you have a good thing running, why stop it? You can choose your ingredients wisely to avoid weight loss and gain muscle mass, as the sirtfood diet can allow you this option as well.

I've just finished phase 2. Do I need to stop drinking the green juice?

Short answer: no. You can still have your morning green juice, as this powerful morning cocktail is the magic potion that can boost the productivity of the sirtuin-activating nutrients. If you want to benefit from the consumption of sirtfoods, you should never stop drinking the morning green juice.

Is it OK to follow this diet if I take medication?

The sirtfood diet can be tried by mostly everyone, but there are a few exceptions. When you are sick and on medication, nutrient deprivation is not something that you need, plus the sirtfood diet can mess with the medication you are taking.

Can children try this diet?

The sirtfood diet was designed to be enjoyed by most of the family, including children. If you have the chance to keep your children away from junk food, why shouldn't you let them reap the benefits of sirtfoods? Obviously, you don't want your children to be hooked on coffee and green tea, and obviously not on red wine. But most of the other ingredients can be tried by children.

Glossary

Antioxidant (dietary) A substance, either human-made or found naturally in food, that, when consumed, reduces the physical stress on the cells in our bodies.

Blue Zones Select geographical regions of the world where people eat diets rich in Sirtfoods and live extraordinarily long, healthy, and happy lives.

Caloric restriction A dietary regimen where people purposely reduce their food intake in an attempt to lose weight, improve health, and extend life span.

DHA (Docosahexaenoic acid) One of two crucial omega-3 fatty acids (alongside EPA), primarily found in oily fish and marine plants like algae, that enhances the activity of our sirtuins and improves overall health.

EPA (Eicosapentaenoic acid) One of two crucial omega-3 fatty acids (alongside DHA), primarily found in oily fish, that enhances the activity of our sirtuins and improves overall health.

Gene Made up of DNA, the blueprint of our bodies; when activated, a gene signals our bodies to produce protein, which changes how our cells work.

Inflammaging A persistent low-grade inflammation that occurs with aging and increases our risk of many chronic diseases.

Leucine An essential amino acid found in dietary protein. It has a potent effect in enhancing the benefits of Sirtfoods, so a Sirtfood diet should also be protein-rich.

Metabolism All the biochemical reactions taking place within a cell that help maintain life.

Mitochondria Tiny structures within a cell that break down nutrients and generate energy. The power the cell to carry out its functions. Muscle cells require a lot of energy, and so are particularly rich in mitochondria.

Polyphenols a large group of natural chemicals found in plants that are part of a plant's defenses against environmental stresses. Certain polyphenols switch on our sirtuin genes when consumed, and give rise to the many benefits of the Sirtfood Diet.

SIRT1 The most thoroughly researched of the sirtuin family of genes and the most important for targeting weight loss. It is activated when cells are stressed and have numerous health and anti-aging effects.

Sirtfood A food particularly rich in specific polyphenols that, when we consume them, can activate our sirtuin genes.

Sirtuin, an ancient family of genes that exist in all of us that are activated when our cells are put under stress. Sirtuins play an essential role in health, disease prevention, and aging. In humans, there are seven different sirtuins (SIRT1 to SIRT7). Of these, SIRT1 and SIRT3 are the two most important sirtuins involved in energy balance.

Stem cell A particular type of cell that can grow into any type of cell found in the body.

Western diet the typical diet representative of industrialized, modern eating patterns and the antithesis of the Blue Zones. A Western diet is characterized by high consumption of processed and refined foods and a notable lack of nutrient-rich plants, especially Sirtfoods.

Conclusion

This ends our book. The Sirt Food diet is a type of diet, and it undoubtedly has significant advantages, it can make you lose weight, maintain muscle mass and promote anti-aging. Sirtfoods are easy to make – they do not require any particular skill before you prepare them. As we can see, many celebrities have undergone this diet, showing that the diet does not require much time.

We neither need to starve ourselves nor need to wage war against food before we get the heavenly body we crave for. We need to ask questions like, "Why do people feel that they need to eat, why do they feel like they will die if they do not eat at least three times a day, why do they feel they are performing some kind of sacrifice if anytime they don't eat?". We also do not need to question the importance of food because food is undisputedly essential. We have to strictly adhere to the laid down instructions and suggestions made by the renowned nutritionist that made sirtfood diet known to the world.

It is time people should eventually realize that they need not starve themselves before they can lose weight. All they need is to diet in sirtfoods, which has recently been proven to be a very effective way of losing weight and shedding fat while gaining muscle at the same time. Sirtfood diets have quite several advantages over all other diets. It is imperative to get ourselves informed that sirtfoods are full of healthy food, but it is not an entirely healthy eating pattern.

We do not need to become extremists, all in the name of losing weight. Too much exercise, just like any other thing in the universe, is hazardous to our health. It can cause hormonal disorder, which might even lead to obesity (if testosterone is affected). It can lead to fatigue when cortisol, the stress hormone is altered; it can easily strain one's body and get injured; it can also lead to overeating. In this situation, the body starts to burn muscle instead of fat.

That is why have everything in moderation, especially when you just finished phase 1 and 2 of this diet. Take everything slowly and always listen to your body.

Although the early stage of juicing and fasting is ideal for those who might want to lose a little weight rapidly, the Sirtfood diet's overall goal is to include nutritious foods in your diet to improve your well-being and immune system. There's one more important goal, though. Although the first seven days can sound very challenging, the longer-term approach will work for everybody.

You will start the fat burning while enjoying your daily favorites by concentrating on incorporating Sirtfood rich ingredients into your everyday meals. It is an eating program and will continue to provide results for a long period.

All this being said, we can easily finalize that sirtfoods diet is the best diet in the universe now. It is easy and natural to do, it does not require extreme exercise, and it does not require starvation of the person dieting. These are just one of the reasons we have to admit that no other diet can be compared to the sirtfood diet in recent years.

The Sirt Food Diet helps us to continue eating many foods, which in other diet forbids. However, this does not mean being able to eat without control. Indeed, we must follow a very strict protocol. With this, I do not want to discourage you, but only to make you realize that there are other ways, which can lead to equally valid results. It should be stressed, however, that the Sirt Food diet is considered safe, the side effects are minimal and temporary.

I hope you learned a lot of information as you start your journey with Sirtfood Diet.

Thank you!
Amy Cook